BELIEVE IT OR NOT . . . .

* One cigarette destroys 25 mg of vitamin C.
* Lecithin can provide the same stick-free pots and pans that Pam does—without propellents!
* Milk with synthetic vitamin D can rob the body of magnesium!
* People who live in smoggy cities are not getting the vitamin D that their country cousins get because the smog absorbs the sun's ultraviolet rays!
* More than one cocktail a day can cause a depletion of vitamins B_1, B_6 and folic acid!
* Oral contraceptives (The Pill) can interfere with the availability of vitamins B_6, B_{12}, folic acid and vitamin C!
* Cancer researchers at the Massachusetts Institute of Technology have found that vitamins C and E and certain chemicals called indoles, found in cabbage, Brussels sprouts, and related vegetables in the crucifer family, are potent and safe inhibitors of certain carcinogens.
* Vitamin B_1 can help fight air and seasickness.
* If you're on a high-protein diet your need for B_6 *increases*.

IT'S ALL HERE AND MUCH MORE IN
EARL MINDELL'S
~~VITAMIN BIBLE~~

Times

*How the Right Vitamins
& Nutrient Supplements Can Help
Turn Your Life Around*

EARL MINDELL'S VITAMIN BIBLE

EARL MINDELL

WARNER BOOKS

A Warner Communications Company

This Book is dedicated to
GAIL, ALANNA, EVAN,

our parents and families

and to
the future

WARNER BOOKS EDITION

Copyright © 1979 by Earl Mindell and Hester Mundis
All rights reserved.

This Warner Books Edition is published by arrangement with
Rawson Associates,
597 Fifth Avenue,
New York, N.Y. 10017

Warner Books, Inc.
666 Fifth Avenue
New York, N.Y. 10103

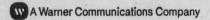 A Warner Communications Company

Printed in the United States of America

First Warner Books Printing: January, 1981

35   34

The first wealth is health.

Ralph Waldo Emerson
"The Conduct of Life"

Acknowledgments

I wish to express my deep and lasting appreciation to my friends and associates who have assisted me in the preparation of this book, especially J. Kenney, Ph.D.; Linus Pauling, Ph.D.; Hester Mundis; Bernard Bubman, R.Ph.; and Mel Rich, R.Ph.

I would also like to thank the Nutrition Foundation; the International College of Applied Nutrition; the American Medical Association; the New York Blood Center; the American Academy of Pediatrics; the American Dietetic Association; the National Academy of Sciences; the National Dairy Council; the Society for Nutrition Education; the United Fresh Fruit and Vegetable Association; the Albany College of Pharmacy; Peter Mallory; Edward Leavitt, D.V.M.; Debbi Quick; Ronald Borenstein; Laura Borenstein; Martha Millard and Richard Curtis, without whom a project of this scope could never have been completed.

Preface

This book is written for *you*—the untold legions of men and women who are forever trying to fit yourselves into statistical norms only to find that the charts are designed for some mythical average person who is taller, shorter, fatter, skinnier, less or more active than you'll ever be. It is a guide to healthy living for individuals, not statistics. Wherever feasible I have given personal advice, for this, I believe, is the only way to lead anyone to optimal health, which is the purpose of this book.

In these pages I have combined my knowledge of pharmacy with that of nutrition to best explain the confusing, often dangerous, interrelation of drugs and vitamins. I've attempted to personalize and be specific so as to eliminate much of the confusion about vitamins that has arisen with generalizations.

In using the book you will occasionally find that your vitamin needs fall into several different categories. In this case, let common sense dictate the necessary adjustment. (If you are already taking B$_6$, for example, there's no need to double up on it unless a higher dosage is called for.)

The recommendations I've made are not meant to be prescriptive, but can easily be used as flexible programs when working with your doctor. No book can substitute for professional care.

It is my sincerest hope that I have provided you with information that will help you attain the longest, happiest, and healthiest of lives.

EARL MINDELL, *Pharm.B., R.Ph.*

Contents

PART ONE

THE WHOLE TRUTH

I. Getting into Vitamins   19

(1) Why I did—(2) What vitamins are—(3) What
vitamins are not—(4) How they work—(5) Should
you take supplements?—(6) What are nutrients?—(7)
The difference between micronutrients and macro-
nutrients—(8) How nutrients get to work—(9) Understanding your digestive system—(10) Name that
vitamin—(11) Name that mineral—(12) Your body
needs togetherness—(13) Eye-opening vitamin facts

II. A Vitamin Pill Is a Vitamin Pill Is a . . .

35

(14) Where vitamins come from—(15) Why vitamins
come in different forms—(16) Oil vs. dry or water
soluble—(17) Synthetic vs. natural and inorganic vs.
organic—(18) Chelation, and what it means—(19)
Time release—(20) Fillers, binders, or what else am
I getting?—(21) Storage and staying power—(22)
When and how to take supplements—(23) What's
right for you

PART THREE

VITAMINS VS. DRUGS

PART ONE
THE WHOLE TRUTH

I

Getting into Vitamins

1. Why I Did

My professional education was strictly establishment when it came to vitamins. My courses in pharmacology, biochemistry, organic and inorganic chemistry, and public health hardly dealt with vitamins at all—except in relation to deficiency diseases. Lack of vitamin C? Scurvy. Out of B_1? Beriberi. Not enough vitamin D? Rickets. My courses were the standard fare, with the usual references to a balanced diet and eating the "right foods" (all unappetizingly illustrated on semiglossy charts).

There were no references to vitamins being used for disease prevention or as ways to optimum health.

> Both of us were working fifteen hours
> a day, but only *I* looked and felt it.

In 1965 I opened my first pharmacy. Until then I never realized just how many drugs people were taking, not for illness but simply to get through the day. (I had one regular patron who had prescriptions for pills to supplant virtually all his bodily functions—and he wasn't even sick!) My partner at the time was very vitamin-oriented. Both of us were working fifteen hours a day, but only *I* looked and felt it. When I asked him what his secret was, he said it was no secret at all. It was vitamins. I realized what he was talking about had very little to do with scurvy and beriberi and a lot to do with me. I instantly became an eager pupil, and have never since regretted it. He taught me the benefits that could be reaped from nature's own foods in the form of vitamins, how B complex and C could alleviate stress, how vitamin E would increase my endurance and stamina, and how B_{12} could eliminate fatigue. After embarking on the most elementary vitamin regimens I was not only convinced. I was converted.

Suddenly nutrition became the most important thing in my life. I read every book I could find on the subject, clipped articles and tracked down their sources, dug out my pharmacy school texts and discovered the amazingly close relationship that did exist between biochemistry and nutrition. I attended any health lecture I could. (It was at one such lecture that I learned of the RNA-DNA nucleic complex and its age-reversing properties. I have been taking RNA-

DNA supplements since then, and today most people guess me to be five to ten years younger than I am.) I was excited about each new discovery in the field, and it showed.

A whole new world had opened up for me and I wanted others to share it. My partner understood completely. We began giving out samples of B complex and B_{12} tablets to patrons, suggesting they try decreasing their dependency on tranquilizers, pep pills, and sedatives with the vitamins and vitamin-rich foods.

The results were remarkable! People kept coming back to tell us how much better and more energetic they felt. Instead of the negativity and resignation that often accompanies drug therapies, we received overwhelming positiveness. I saw a woman who had spent nearly all her young adult life on Librium, running from doctor to therapist and back again, become a healthy, happy, drug-free human being; a sixty-year-old architect, on the brink of retirement because of ill health, regain his well-being and accept a commission for what is now one of the foremost office buildings in Los Angeles; a middle-aged pill-dependent actor kick his habit and land a sought-after supporting role in a TV series that still nets him handsome residuals.

By 1970 I was totally committed to nutrition and preventive medicine. Seeing the paucity of knowledge in the area, I went into partnership with another pharmacist for the prime purpose of making natural vitamins and accurate nutrition information available to the public.

Today, as a nutritionist, lecturer, and author, I'm still excited about that world that opened

21

up to me over fifteen years ago—a world that continues to grow with new discoveries daily—and I'm eager to share it.

2. What Vitamins Are

> We must obtain vitamins from organic foods, or dietary supplements in order to sustain life.

When I mention the word "vitamin," most people think "pill." Thinking "pill" brings to mind confusing images of medicine and drugs. Though vitamins can and certainly often do the work of both medicine and drugs, they are neither.

• Quite simply, vitamins are organic substances necessary for life. Vitamins are essential to the normal functioning of our bodies and, save for a few exceptions, cannot be manufactured or synthesized by our bodies. They are necessary for our growth, vitality, and general well-being. In their natural state they are found in minute quantities in all organic food. We must obtain them from these foods or in dietary supplements.

Supplements, which usually come in pill form and around which so much controversy has arisen, are still just food substances, and, unless synthetic, are also derived from living plants and animals.

• It is impossible to sustain life without *all* the essential vitamins.

3. What Vitamins Are Not

> Vitamins are neither pep pills nor
> substitutes for food.

A lot of people think vitamins can replace food. They cannot. In fact, vitamins cannot be assimilated without ingesting food. There are a lot of erroneous beliefs about vitamins, and I hope this book can clear up most of them.

• Vitamins are not pep pills and have no caloric or energy value of their own.
• Vitamins are not substitutes for protein or for any other nutrients, such as minerals, fats, carbohydrates, water—or even for each other!
• Vitamins themselves are not the components of our body structures.
• You cannot take vitamins, stop eating, and expect to be healthy.

4. How They Work

If you think of the body as an automobile's combustion engine and vitamins as spark plugs, you have a fairly good idea of how these amazing minute food substances work for us.

> Vitamins regulate our metabolism through
> enzyme systems. A single deficiency can
> endanger the whole body.

Vitamins are components of our enzyme systems which, acting like spark plugs, energize and regulate our metabolism, keeping us tuned up and functioning at high performance.

Compared with our intake of other nutrients like proteins, fats, and carbohydrates, our vitamin intake (even on some megadose regimens) is minuscule. But a deficiency in even one vitamin can endanger the whole human body.

5. Should You Take Supplements?

> "Everyone who has in the past eaten sugar, white flour, or canned food has some deficiency disease. . . ."

Since vitamins occur in all organic material, some containing more of one vitamin than another and in greater or lesser amounts, you could say that if you ate the "right" foods in a well-balanced diet, you would get all the vitamins you need. And you would probably be right. The problem is, very few of us are able to arrange this mythical diet. According to Dr. Daniel T. Quigley, author of *The National Malnutrition,* "Everyone who has in the past eaten sugar, white flour, or canned food has some deficiency disease, the extent of the disease depending on the percentage of such deficient food in the diet."

Most of the foods we eat have been processed and depleted in nutrients. Take breads and cereals, for example. Practically all of them you find in today's supermarkets are high in nothing but carbohydrates. "But they are enriched!" you say. It says so right on the label. *Enriched.*

Enriched? The standard of enrichment for white flour is to replace the twenty-two natural nutrients that are removed with three B vitamins, vitamin D, calcium, and iron salts.

• For the staff of life, that seems a pretty flimsy stick. I think the answer on supplements is clear.

6. What Are Nutrients?

They're more than vitamins, though people often think they are the same thing.

Six important nutrients

Carbohydrates, proteins, fats, minerals, vitamins, and water are all nutrients—absorbable components of foods—and necessary for good health. Nutrients are necessary for energy, organ function, food utilization, and cell growth.

7. The Difference Between Micronutrients and Macronutrients

Micronutrients, like vitamins and minerals, do not themselves provide energy. The macronutrients—carbohydrates, fat, and protein—do that, but only when there are sufficient micronutrients to release them.

With nutrients, *less* is often the
same as *more*.

The amount of micronutrients and macro-nutrients you need for proper health is vastly different—but each is important.

8. How Nutrients Get to Work

> The body simplifies nutrients in order to utilize them.

Nutrients basically work through digestion. Digestion is a process of continuous chemical simplification of materials that enter the body through the mouth. Materials are split by enzymatic action into smaller and simpler chemical fragments, which can then be absorbed through walls of the digestive tract—an open-ended muscular tube, more than thirty feet long, which passes through the body—and finally enter the bloodstream.

9. Understanding Your Digestive System

Knowing how your digestive system works will clear up, right at the start, some of the more common confusions about how, when, and where nutrients operate.

Mouth and Esophagus

Digestion begins in the mouth with the grinding of food and admixture of saliva. An enzyme called ptyalin in the saliva already begins to split starches into simple sugars. The food is then forced to the back of the mouth and into the esophagus, or gullet. Here is where peristalsis begins. This is a kneading "milking" constriction and relaxation of muscles that propels material through the digestive system. To prevent backflow of materials, and to time the release of proper enzymes—since one enzyme cannot do another enzyme's work—the digestive tract is equipped with valves at important junctions.

Stomach

This is the biggest bulge in the digestive tract, as most of us are well aware. But it is located higher than you might think, lying mainly behind the lower ribs, not under the navel, and it does not occupy the belly. It is a flexible bag enclosed by restless muscles, constantly changing form.

• Virtually nothing is absorbed through the stomach walls except alcohol.

An ordinary meal leaves the stomach
in three to five hours.

Watery substances, such as soup, leave the stomach quite rapidly. Fats remain considerably longer. An ordinary meal of carbohydrates, proteins, and fats is emptied from the average stomach in *three* to *five* hours. Stomach glands and specialized cells produce mucus, enzymes, hydrochloric acid, and a factor that enables vitamin B_{12} to be dissolved through intestinal walls into the circulation. A normal stomach is

27

definitely on the acid side, and gastric juice, the stomach's special blend, consists of many substances:

Pepsin The predominant stomach enzyme, a potent digester of meats and other proteins. It is active only in an acid medium.
Renin Curdles milk.
HCl (*Hydrochloric acid*) Produced by stomach cells and creates an acidic state.

The stomach is not absolutely indispensable to digestion. Most of the process of digestion occurs beyond it.

Small Intestine

> Virtually all absorption of nutrients occurs in the small intestine.

Twenty-two feet long, here is where digestion is completed and virtually all absorption of nutrients occurs. It has an alkaline environment, brought about by highly alkaline bile, pancreatic juice, and secretions of the intestinal walls. The alkaline environment is necessary for the most important work of digestion and absorption. The *duodenum,* which begins at the stomach outlet, is the first part of the small intestine. This joins with the *jejunum* (about ten feet long), which joins with the *ileum* (ten to twelve feet long). When semiliquid contents of the small intestine are moved along by peristaltic action, we often say we hear our stomach "talking." Actually our stomach lies above these rumblings (called borborygmi), but even with the truth known it's doubtful the phrase will change.

Large Intestine (Colon)

> It takes twelve to fourteen hours for contents to make the circuit of the large intestine.

Any material leaving the ileum and entering the cecum (where the small and large intestines join) is quite watery. Backflow is prevented at this junction by a muscular valve.

Very little is absorbed from the large intestine except water.

The colon is primarily a storage and dehydrating organ. Substances entering in a liquid state become semisolid as water is absorbed. It takes twelve to fourteen hours for contents to make the circuit of the intestine.

The colon, in contrast to the germ-free stomach, is lavishly populated with bacteria, normal intestinal flora. A large part of the feces is composed of bacteria, along with indigestible material, chiefly cellulose, and substances eliminated from the blood and shed from the intestinal walls.

Liver

> The main storage organ for fat-soluble vitamins

The liver is the largest solid organ of the body and weighs about four pounds. It is an incomparable chemical plant. It can modify almost any chemical structure. It is a powerful detoxifying organ, breaking down a variety of toxic molecules and rendering them harmless. It is also a blood reservoir and a storage organ for vitamins such as A and D and for digested carbohydrate (glycogen), which is released to sustain blood sugar levels. It manufactures enzymes, cholesterol, proteins, vitamin A (from carotene), and blood coagulation factors.

One of the prime functions of the liver is to produce bile. Bile contains salts that promote efficient digestion of fats by detergent action, emulsifying fatty materials.

Gallbladder

> Even the sight of food may empty the gallbladder.

This is a saclike storage organ about three inches long. It holds bile, modifies it chemically, and concentrates it tenfold. The taste or sometimes even the sight of food may be sufficient to empty it out. Constituents of gallbladder fluids sometimes crystallize and form gallstones.

Pancreas

> The pancreas provides the body's most important enzymes.

This gland is about six inches long and is nestled into the curve of the duodenum. Its cell clusters secrete insulin, which accelerates the burning of sugar in the body. Insulin is secreted into the blood, not the digestive tract. The larger part of the pancreas manufactures and secretes pancreatic juice, which contains some of the body's most important digestive enzymes—*lipases*, which split fats; *proteases*, which split protein; and *amylases*, which split starches.

10. Name That Vitamin

Because at one time no one knew the chemical structure of vitamins and therefore could not give them a proper scientific name, most are designated by a letter of the alphabet. The following vitamins are known today; many more

```
Known vitamins from A to U
```

have yet to be discovered. A (retinol, carotene); B-complex group: B_1 (thiamine), B_2 (riboflavin), B_3 (niacin, niacinamide), B_5 (pantothenic acid), B_6 (pyridoxine), B_{10}, B_{11}, (growth factors), B_{12} (cobalamin, cyanocobalamin), B_{13} (orotic acid), B_{15} (pangamic acid), B_{17} (amygdalin); PABA (para-aminobenzoic acid); choline; inositol; C (ascorbic acid); D (calciferol, viosterol, ergosterol); E (tocopherol); F (fatty acids); G (riboflavin); H (biotin); K (menadione); L (necessary for lactation); M (folic acid); P (bioflavonoids); T (growth-promoting substances); U (extracted from cabbage juice).

11. Name That Mineral

> The top six minerals are: calcium, iodine, iron, magnesium, phosphorus, and zinc.

Although about eighteen known minerals are required for body maintenance and regulatory functions, Recommended Daily Dietary Allowances (RDA) have only been established for six—calcium, iodine, iron, magnesium, phosphorus, and zinc. (See section 81.)

The active minerals in your body are: calcium, chlorine, chromium, cobalt, copper, fluorine, iodine, iron, magnesium, manganese, molybdenum, phosphorus, potassium, selenium, sodium, sulfur, vanadium, and zinc.

12. Your Body Needs Togetherness

> Vitamins alone are not enough.

As important as vitamins are, they can do nothing for you without minerals. I like to call minerals the Cinderellas of the nutrition world, because, though very few people are aware of it, vitamins cannot function, cannot be assimilated, without the aid of minerals. And though the body can synthesize some vitamins, it cannot manufacture a *single* mineral.

13. Eye-opening Vitamin Facts

Would you believe that...

- One cigarette destroys 25 mg. of vitamin C.
- Lecithin can provide the same stick-free pots and pans that commercially marketed Pam does—and without propellents! (Just break open a lecithin capsule and see for yourself, or check the ingredients on the next can of Pam that you buy.)
- Milk with synthetic vitamin D (which means almost all store-bought milk) can rob the body of magnesium!
- People who live in smoggy cities are not getting the vitamin D that their country cousins get because the smog absorbs the sun's ultraviolet rays!
- Daily "happy hours" of more than one cocktail can cause a depletion of vitamins B_1, B_6, and folic acid!
- Ten million American women take oral contraceptives and most of them are unaware that the pills can interfere with the availability of vitamins B_6, B_{12}, folic acid, and vitamin C!
- American men rank thirteenth in world health, American women sixth.
- Cancer researchers at the Massachusetts Institute of Technology have found that vitamins C and E and certain chemicals called indoles, found in cabbage, Brussels sprouts, and related vegetables in the crucifer family, are potent and

apparently safe inhibitors of certain carcinogens.

• Vitamin B_1 can help fight air and seasickness.

• If you're on a high-protein diet your need for B_6 *increases*.

• The Russians have found that vitamin B_{12} can ward off hangovers.

• Eighteen pecan halves can furnish a day's supply of vitamin F.

II

A Vitamin Pill
Is a Vitamin Pill Is a . . .

14. Where Vitamins Come From

Most vitamins are extracted from
basic natural sources.

Because vitamins are natural substances found
in foods, the supplements you take—be they
capsules, tablets, powders, or liquids—also
come from foods. Though many of the vitamins
can be synthesized, most are extracted from
basic natural sources.

For example: Vitamin A usually comes from
fish liver oil. Vitamin B complex comes from
yeast or liver. Vitamin C is best when derived
from rose hips, the berries found on the fruit
of the rose after the petals have fallen off. And

vitamin E is generally extracted from soybeans, wheat germ, or corn.

15. Why Vitamins Come in Different Forms

Everyone's needs are different, and for this reason manufacturers have provided many vitamins in a variety of forms.

> Vitamins come in different forms
> because people do.

Tablets are the most common and convenient form. They're easier to store, carry, and have a longer shelf life than powders or liquids.

Capsules, like tablets, are convenient and easy to store, and are the usual supplement for oil-soluble vitamins such as A, D, and E.

Powders have advantages of extra potency (1 tsp. of many vitamin-C powders can give you as much as 4,000 mg.) and the added benefit of no fillers, binders, or additives for anyone with allergies.

Liquids are available for easy mixing with beverages and for people unable to swallow capsules and tablets.

16. Oil vs. Dry or Water Soluble

The oil-soluble vitamins, such as A, D, and E, are available and advisable in "dry" or water-soluble form for people who tend to get upset stomaches from oil, for acne sufferers, or anyone with a skin condition where oil ingestion is not advised, and for dieters who have cut most of the fat from their meals. (Fat-soluble vitamins need fat for proper assimilation. If you're on a low-fat diet and taking A, D, or E supplements, I suggest you use the dry form.)

17. Synthetic vs. Natural and Inorganic vs. Organic

> Synthetic vitamins can cause toxic reactions, while natural vitamins, even with high doses, don't.

When I'm asked if there's a difference between synthetic and natural vitamins, I usually say only one—and that's to you. Though synthetic vitamins and minerals have produced satisfactory results, the benefits from natural vitamins, on a variety of levels, surpass them. Chemical analysis of both might appear the same, but there's more to natural vitamins because there's more to those substances in nature.

Synthetic vitamin C is just that, ascorbic acid and nothing more. Natural vitamin C from rose hips contains bioflavonoids, the entire C complex, which make the C much more effective.

Natural vitamin E, which can include all the tocopherals, not just alpha, is more potent than its synthetic double.

According to Dr. Theron G. Randolph, noted allergist:

A synthetically derived substance may cause a reaction in a chemically susceptible person when the same material of natural origin is tolerated, despite the two substances having identical chemical structures.

And as many who have tried both can attest, there are less gastrointestinal upsets with natural supplements. Also, and perhaps most important, synthetic vitamins can cause toxic reactions, while these reactions don't occur with natural vitamins when taken in higher than usual dosage.

The difference between inorganic and organic is not the same as the one between synthetic and natural, though that is the common misconception. All vitamins are organic. They are substances containing carbon.

Minerals, however, are inorganic. They do not contain carbon. But there are organic irons —ferrous gluconate, ferrous peptonate, and ferrous citrate. Ferrous sulfate, on the other hand, is an inorganic iron.

18. Chelation, and What It Means

Only 2 to 10 percent of inorganic iron taken into the body is actually absorbed.

First, pronounce it correctly. *Key' lation.* This is the process by which mineral substances are changed into their digestible form. Common mineral supplements such as bonemeal and dolomite are often not chelated and must first be acted upon in the digestive process to form chelates before they are of use to the body. The natural chelating process is not performed efficiently in many people, and because of this a good deal of the mineral supplements they take is of little use.

When you realize that the body does not use whatever it takes in, that most of us do not digest our foods efficiently, that only 2 to 10 percent of inorganic iron taken into the body is actually absorbed, and, even with this small percentage, 50 percent is then eliminated, you can recognize the importance of taking minerals that have been chelated. Chelated mineral supplements provide three to ten times greater assimilation than the nonchelated ones, and are well worth the small additional cost.

19. Time Release

A major step forward in vitamin manufacturing has been the introduction of time-release supplements. Time release is a process by which vitamins are enrobed in micropellets (tiny time pills) and then combined into a special base for their release in a pattern that assures eight- to twelve-hour absorption. Most vitamins are water soluble and cannot be stored in the body. Without time release, they are quickly absorbed into the bloodstream, and, no matter how large the dose, are excreted in the urine within two to three hours.

A way to twenty-four-hour vitamin
protection.

Time-release supplements can offer optimum effectiveness, minimal excretary loss, and stable blood levels all during the day and through the night.

20. Fillers, Binders, Or What Else Am I Getting?

There's more to a vitamin supplement than meets the eye—and sometimes more than meets the label. Fillers, binders, lubricants, and the like do not have to be listed and often aren't. But if you'd like to know what you're swallowing, the following list should help.

Diluents or fillers These are inert materials added to the tablets to increase their bulk, in order to make them a practical size for compression. Dicalcium phosphate, which is an excellent source of calcium and phosphorus, is used in better brands. It is derived from purified mineral rocks. It is a white powder. Sorbitol and cellulose (plant fiber) are used occasionally.

Binders These substances give cohesive qualities to the powdered materials, otherwise the binders or granulators are the materials that hold the ingredients of the tablet together. Cellulose and ethyl cellulose are used most often. Cellulose is the main constituent of plant fiber. Other binders that can be used are:

  acacia (gum arabic)—a vegetable gum
  algin—alginic acid or sodium alginate—a plant carbohydrate derived from seaweed
  lecithin and sorbitol are used occasionally

Lubricants A slick substance added to a

tablet to keep it from sticking to the machines that punch it out. Calcium stearate and silica are commonly used. Calcium stearate is derived from natural vegetable oils. Silica is a natural white powder. Magnesium stearate can also be used.

Disintegrators Substances such as gum arabic, algin, and alginate are added to the tablet to facilitate its breakup or disintegration after ingestion.

Colors They make the tablet more esthetic or elegant in appearance. Colors derived from natural sources, like chlorophyll, are best.

Flavors and sweeteners Used only in chewable tablets, the sweeteners are usually fructose (fruit sugar), malt dextrins, sorbitol, or maltose. Sucrose (sugar) is rarely used in better brands.

Coating materials These substances are used to protect the tablet from moisture. They also mask unpleasant flavor or odor and make the tablet easier to swallow. Zein is one of the substances. It is natural, derived from corn protein, and a clear film-coating agent. Brazil Wax, which is a natural product derived from palm trees, is also frequently used.

Drying agents These substances prevent water-absorbing (hydroscopic) materials from picking up moisture during processing. Silica gel is the most common drying agent.

21. Storage and Staying Power

Vitamin and mineral supplements should be stored in a cool dark place away from direct sunlight in a well-closed—preferably opaque—

container. They do not have to be stored in the refrigerator unless you live in a desert climate. To guard against excessive moisture, place a few kernels of rice at the bottom of your vitamin bottle. The rice works as a natural absorbent.

Vitamins can last two to three years
in a well-sealed container.

If vitamins are kept cool and away from light, and remain well sealed, they should last for two to three years. Once a bottle is opened you can expect a twelve-month shelf life.

Our bodies tend to excrete in urine substances we take in on a four-hour basis, and this is particularly true of water-soluble vitamins such as B and C. On an empty stomach, B and C vitamins can leave the body as quickly as two hours after ingestion.

The oil-soluble vitamins, A, D, E, and K, remain in the body for approximately twenty-four hours, though excess amounts can be stored in the liver for much longer. Dry A and E do not stay in the body as long.

22. When and How to Take Supplements

The human body operates on a twenty-four-hour cycle. Your cells do not go to sleep when you do, nor can they exist without continuous oxygen and nutrients. Therefore, for best results, space your supplements as evenly as possible during the day.

> If you take your supplements all
> at once, do so after dinner,
> not breakfast.

The prime time for taking supplements is after meals. Vitamins are organic substances and should be taken with other foods and minerals for best absorption. Because the water-soluble vitamins, especially B complex and C, are excreted fairly rapidly in the urine, a regimen of after breakfast, after lunch, and after dinner will provide you with the highest body level. If after each meal is not convenient, then half the amount should be taken after breakfast and the other half after dinner.

If you must take your vitamins all at once, then do so after the largest meal of the day. In other words, for best results, after dinner, not after breakfast, is the most desirable.

And remember, minerals are essential for proper vitamin absorption, so be sure to take your minerals and vitamins together.

23. What's Right for You

If you're unsure as to whether you'd be better off with a powder, a liquid, or a tablet, regular vitamin E or dry, taking supplements three times a day or time released, my advice to you is to experiment. If the supplement you're taking doesn't agree with you, try it in another form. Vitamin-C powder mixed in a beverage might be much easier to take than several large pills when you're coming down with a cold. If your face breaks out with vitamin E, try the dry form. Check sections 24 through 71 and the cautions in section 98 to make sure you know all you should about your supplement.

III

Everything You Always Wanted to Know About Vitamins but Had No One to Ask

24. Vitamin A

FACTS:

Vitamin A is fat soluble. It requires fats as well as minerals to be properly absorbed by your digestive tract.

It can be stored in your body and need not be replenished every day.

It occurs in two forms—preformed vitamin A, called retinol (found only in foods of animal origin), and provitamin A, known as carotene (provided by foods of both plant and animal origin).

Vitamin A is measured in USP Units (United States Pharmacopea), IU (International Units), and RE (Retinol Equivalents). (See section 80.)

10,000 IU daily is the average adult dosage, though the need increases with greater body weight.

What It Can Do For You:

Counteract night blindness, weak eyesight, and aid in the treatment of many eye disorders. (It permits formation of visual purple in the eye.)

Build resistance to respiratory infections.

Shorten the duration of diseases.

Keep the outer layers of your tissues and organs healthy.

Promote growth, strong bones, healthy skin, hair, teeth, and gums.

Help treat acne, impetigo, boils, carbuncles, and open ulcers when applied externally.

Aid in the treatment of emphysema and hyperthyroidism.

Deficiency Disease:

Xerophthalmia, night blindness. (For deficiency symptoms, see section 76.)

Best Natural Sources:

Fish liver oil, liver, carrots, green and yellow vegetables, eggs, milk and dairy products, margarine, and yellow fruits.

Supplements:

Usually available in two forms, one derived from natural fish liver oil and the other water dispersible. Water-dispersible supplements are either acetate or palmitate and recommended for anyone intolerant to oil, particularly acne sufferers.

Vitamin A acid (retin A) is sometimes prescribed for acne, but is available only by prescription. 10,000 to 25,000 IU are the most common daily doses.

TOXICITY:

More than 100,000 IU daily can produce toxic effects in adults, if taken for many months.

More than 18,500 IU daily can produce toxic effects in infants.

Toxicity symptoms include hair loss, nausea, vomiting, diarrhea, scaly skin, blurred vision, rashes, bone pain, irregular menses, fatigue, headaches, and liver enlargement. (See section 98, "Cautions.")

ENEMIES:

Polyunsaturated fatty acids with carotene work against vitamin A unless there are antioxidants present. (See section 195 for antioxidants, and section 206 for drugs that deplete vitamins.)

PERSONAL ADVICE:

You need at least 10,000 IU vitamin A if you take more than 400 IU vitamin E daily.

If you are on the pill, your need for A is *decreased*.

If your weekly diet includes ample amounts of liver, carrots, spinach, sweet potatoes, or cantaloupe, it's unlikely you need an A supplement.

Do not supplement your dog's or cat's diet with vitamin A unless a vet specifically advises it. (See section 98.)

25. Vitamin B₁ (Thiamine)

FACTS:

Water soluble. Like all the B-complex vitamins, any excess is excreted and not stored in the body. It must be replaced daily.

Measured in milligrams (mg.).

B vitamins are synergistic—they are more potent together than when used separately. B_1, B_2, and B_6 should be equally balanced (i.e., 50 mg. of B_1, 50 mg. of B_2, and 50 mg. of B_6) to work effectively.

The official RDA for adults is 1.2 to 1.4 mg. (During pregnancy and lactation 1.4 mg. is suggested.)

Need increases during illness, stress, and surgery.

Known as the "morale vitamin" because of its beneficial effects on the nervous system and mental attitude.

Has a mild diuretic effect.

WHAT IT CAN DO FOR YOU:

Promote growth.

Aid digestion, especially of carbohydrates.

Improve your mental attitude.

Keep nervous system, muscles, and heart functioning normally.

Help fight air or seasickness.

Relieve dental postoperative pain.

Aid in treatment of herpes zoster.

DEFICIENCY DISEASE:

Beriberi. (For deficiency symptoms, see section 76.)

BEST NATURAL SOURCES:

Dried yeast, rice husks, whole wheat, oatmeal, peanuts, pork, most vegetables, bran, milk.

SUPPLEMENTS:

Available in low- and high-potency dosages —usually 50 mg., 100 mg., and 500 mg. It is most effective in B-complex formulas, balanced with B_2 and B_6. It is even more effective when the formula contains antistress pantothenic acid, folic acid, and B_{12}. 100 to 300 mg. are the most common daily doses.

TOXICITY:

No known toxicity for this water-soluble vitamin. Any excess is excreted in the urine and not stored to any degree in tissues or organs.

Rare excess symptoms include tremors, herpes, edema, nervousness, rapid heartbeat, and allergies.

ENEMIES:

Cooking heat easily destroys this B vitamin. Other enemies of B_1 are caffeine, alcohol, food-processing methods, air, water, estrogen, and sulfa drugs. (See section 206 for drugs that deplete vitamin.)

If you are a smoker, drinker, or heavy sugar consumer, you need more vitamin B_1.

If you are pregnant, nursing, or on the pill you have a greater need for this vitamin.

As with all stress conditions—disease, anxiety, trauma, postsurgery—your B-complex intake, which includes thiamine, should be increased.

26. Vitamin B_2 (Riboflavin)

Facts:

Water soluble. Easily absorbed. The amount excreted depends on bodily needs and may be accompanied by protein loss. Like the other B vitamins it is not stored and must be replaced regularly through whole foods or supplements.

Also known as vitamin G.

Measured in milligrams (mg.).

Unlike thiamine, riboflavin is *not* destroyed by heat, oxidation, or acid.

For normal adults, 1.2 to 1.6 mg. is the RDA. Slightly higher amounts are suggested during pregnancy and lactation.

Increased need in stress situations.

America's most common vitamin deficiency is riboflavin.

What It Can Do For You:

Aid in growth and reproduction.
Promote healthy skin, nails, hair.
Help eliminate sore mouth, lips, and tongue.
Benefit vision, alleviate eye fatigue.

Function with other substances to metabolize carbohydrates, fats, and proteins.

Deficiency Disease:

Ariboflavinosis—mouth, lips, skin, genitalia lesions. (For deficiency symptoms, see section 76.)

Best Natural Sources:

Milk, liver, kidney, yeast, cheese, leafy green vegetables, fish, eggs.

Supplements:

Available in both low and high potencies—most commonly in 100-mg. doses. Like most of the B-complex vitamins, it is most effective when in a well-balanced formula with the others.

100 to 300 mg. are the most common daily doses.

Toxicity:

No known toxic effects.

Possible symptoms of minor excess include itching, numbness, sensations of burning or prickling.

Enemies:

Light—especially ultraviolet light—and alkalies are destructive to riboflavin. (Opaque milk cartons now protect riboflavin that used to be destroyed in clear glass milk bottles.) Other natural enemies are water (B_2 dissolves in cooking liquids), sulfa drugs, estrogen, alcohol. (See section 206.)

If you are taking the pill, pregnant, or lactating, you need more vitamin B₂.

If you eat little red meat or dairy products you should increase your intake.

There is a strong likelihood of your being deficient in this vitamin if you are on a prolonged restricted diet for ulcers or diabetes. (In all cases where you are under medical treatment for a specific illness, check with your doctor before altering your present food regimen or embarking on a new one.)

All stress conditions require additional B complex.

27. Vitamin B₆ (Pyridoxine)

FACTS:

Water soluble. Excreted within eight hours after ingestion and, like the other B vitamins, needs to be replaced by whole foods or supplements.

B₆ is actually a group of substances—pyridoxine, pyridoxinal, and pyridoxamine—that are closely related and function together.

Measured in milligrams (mg.).

Requirement increased when high-protein diets are consumed.

Must be present for the production of antibodies and red blood cells.

There is some evidence of synthesis by intestinal bacteria, and that a vegetable diet supplemented with cellulose is responsible.

The recommended adult intake is 1.6 to 2.0 mg. daily, with higher doses suggested during pregnancy and lactation.

Required for the proper absorption of vitamin B_{12}.

Necessary for the production of hydrochloric acid and magnesium.

WHAT IT CAN DO FOR YOU:

Properly assimilate protein and fat.

Aid in the conversion of tryptophan, an essential amino acid, to niacin.

Help prevent various nervous and skin disorders.

Alleviate nausea (many morning-sickness preparations that doctors prescribe include vitamin B_6).

Promote proper synthesis of antiaging nucleic acids.

Reduce night muscle spasms, leg cramps, hand numbness, certain forms of neuritis in the extremities.

Work as a natural diuretic.

DEFICIENCY DISEASE:

Anemia, seborrheic dermatitis, glossitis. (For deficiency symptoms, see section 76.)

BEST NATURAL SOURCES:

Brewer's yeast, wheat bran, wheat germ, liver, kidney, heart, cantaloupe, cabbage, blackstrap molasses, milk, eggs, beef.

SUPPLEMENTS:

Readily available in a wide range of dosages —from 50 to 500 mg.—in individual supplements as well as in B-complex and multivitamin formulas.

To prevent deficiencies in other B vitamins, pyridoxine should be taken in equal amounts with B_1 and B_2.

Can be purchased in time-disintegrating formulas that provide for gradual release up to ten hours.

TOXICITY:

No known toxic effects.

Possible symptom of an oversupply of B_6 is night restlessness and too vivid dream recall.

ENEMIES:

Long storage, canning, roasting or stewing of meat, water, food-processing techniques, alcohol, estrogen. (See section 206.)

PERSONAL ADVICE:

If you are on the pill, you are more than likely to need increased amounts of B_6.

Heavy protein consumers need extra amounts of this vitamin.

If you are taking a B complex, make sure there is enough B_6 in the formula to be effective. B_6 is expensive, and some vitamin formulas are short on it. If you can't remember your dreams, it might be that you need a separate pyridoxine tablet in addition to your multivitamin or B complex.

28. Vitamin B$_{12}$ (Cobalamin)

FACTS:

Water soluble and effective in very small doses.

Commonly known as the "red vitamin," also cyanocobalamin.

Measured in micrograms (mcg.).

The only vitamin that contains essential mineral elements.

Not well assimilated through the stomach. Needs to be combined with calcium during absorption to properly benefit body.

Recommended adult dose is 3 mcg., with larger amounts suggested for pregnant and lactating women.

A diet low in B$_1$ and high in folic acid (such as a vegetarian diet) often hides a vitamin-B$_{12}$ deficiency.

A properly functioning thyroid gland helps B$_{12}$ absorption. Symptoms of B$_{12}$ deficiency may take more than five years to appear after body stores have been depleted.

WHAT IT CAN DO FOR YOU:

Form and regenerate red blood cells, thereby preventing anemia.

Promote growth and increase appetite in children.

Increase energy.

Maintain a healthy nervous system.

Properly utilize fats, carbohydrates, and protein.

Relieve irritability.

Improve concentration, memory, and balance.

55

DEFICIENCY DISEASE:

Pernicious anemia, brain damage. (For deficiency symptoms, see section 76.)

BEST NATURAL SOURCES:

Liver, beef, pork, eggs, milk, cheese, kidney.

SUPPLEMENTS:

Because B_{12} is not absorbed well through the stomach, I recommend the time-release form of tablet so that it can be assimilated in the small intestine.

Supplements are available in a variety of strengths from 50 mcg. to 2,000 mcg.

Doctors routinely give vitamin-B_{12} injections. If there is a severe indication of deficiency or extreme fatigue, this method might be the supplementation that's called for.

Daily doses most often used are 5 to 100 mcg.

TOXICITY:

There have been no cases reported of vitamin-B_{12} toxicity, even on megadose regimens.

ENEMIES:

Acids and alkalies, water, sunlight, alcohol, estrogen, sleeping pills. (See section 206.)

PERSONAL ADVICE:

If you are a vegetarian and have excluded eggs and dairy products from your diet, then you need B_{12} supplementation.

Combined with folic acid, B_{12} can be a most effective revitalizer.

Surprisingly, heavy protein consumers may also need extra amounts of this vitamin, which works synergistically with almost all other B vitamins as well as vitamins A, E, and C.

Women may find B_{12} helpful—as part of a B complex—during and just prior to menstruation.

29. Vitamin B_{13} (Orotic Acid)

FACTS:

Not yet available in the United States, but can be obtained in Europe.

Metabolizes folic acid and vitamin B_{12}.

No RDA has been established.

WHAT IT CAN DO FOR YOU:

Possibly prevent certain liver problems and premature aging.

Aid in the treatment of multiple sclerosis.

DEFICIENCY DISEASE:

Deficiency symptoms and diseases related to this vitamin are still uncertain.

BEST NATURAL SOURCES:

Root vegetables, whey, the liquid portion of soured or curdled milk.

Available as calcium orotate in supplemental form.

TOXICITY:

Too little is known about the vitamin at this time to establish guidelines.

ENEMIES:

Water and sunlight.

PERSONAL ADVICE:

Not enough research has been done on this vitamin for recommendations to be made.

30. B₁₅ (Pangamic Acid)

FACTS:

Water soluble.
Because its essential requirement for diet has not been proved, it is not a vitamin in the strict sense.
Measured in milligrams (mg.).
Works much like vitamin E in that it is an antioxidant.
Introduced by the Russians, who are thrilled with its results, while the U.S. Food and Drug Administration wants it off the market.
Action is often improved by being taken with vitamins A and E.

What It Can Do For You: *

Extend cell life span.
Neutralize the craving for liquor.
Speed recovery from fatigue.
Lower blood cholesterol levels.
Protect against pollutants.
Aid in protein synthesis.
Relieve symptoms of angina and asthma.
Protect the liver against cirrhosis.
Ward off hangovers.
Stimulate immunity responses.

Deficiency Disease:

Again, research has been limited, but indications point to glandular and nerve disorders, heart disease, and diminished oxygenation of living tissue.

Best Natural Sources:

Brewer's yeast, whole brown rice, whole grains, pumpkin seeds, sesame seeds.

Supplements:

Usually available in 50-mg. strengths.
Daily doses most often used are 50 to 150 mgs.

Toxicity:

There have been no reported cases of toxicity. Some people say they have experienced nausea

*U.S. research in the case of B_{15} has been limited. The list of benefits given here is based on my study of Soviet tests.

on beginning a B_{15} regimen, but this usually disappears after a few days and can be alleviated by taking the B_{15} supplement after the day's largest meal.

ENEMIES:

Water and sunlight.

PERSONAL ADVICE:

Despite the controversy, I have found B_{15} effective and believe most diets would benefit from supplementation.

(Dr. Atkins prescribes it for anyone on his super-energy diet.)

If you are an athlete or just want to feel like one, I suggest one 50-mg. tablet in the morning with breakfast and one in the evening with dinner.

An important supplement for residents of big cities and high-density pollution areas.

31. Vitamin B_{17} (Laetrile)

FACTS:

One of the most controversial "vitamins" of the decade.

Chemically a compound of two sugar molecules (one benzaldehyde and one cyanide) called an amygdalin.

Known as nitrilosides when used in medical doses.

Made from apricot pits.

One B vitamin that is not present in brewer's yeast.

Unaccepted as a cancer treatment in most of the United States at this date. (Legal in fifteen states.) Rejected by the Food and Drug Administration on the grounds it might be poisonous due to its cyanide content.

WHAT IT CAN DO FOR YOU:

It is purported to have specific cancer-controlling and preventive properties.

DEFICIENCY DISEASE:

May lead to diminished resistance to cancer.

BEST NATURAL SOURCES:

A small amount of laetrile is found in the whole kernels of apricots, apples, cherries, peaches, plums, and nectarines.

SUPPLEMENTS:

Daily doses most often used are 0.25 to 1.0 g.

TOXICITY:

Though no toxicity levels have been established yet, taking excessive amounts of laetrile could be dangerous. Cumulative amounts of more than 3.0 g. can be ingested safely, but not more than 1.0 g. at any one time.

According to the *Nutrition Almanac,* five to thirty apricot kernels eaten throughout the day, but never all at the same time, can be a sufficient preventive amount.

If you are interested in laetrile as a cancer preventive or treatment, check with a nutrition-oriented physician. If you know of none in your area, ask the International College of Applied Nutrition (Box 386, La Habra, California 90631) for a referral.

There is now extensive literature available on laetrile. I strongly advise personal research and a consultation with a physician before embarking on any regimen involving B_{17}.

32. Biotin (Coenzyme R or Vitamin H)

FACTS:

Water soluble, and another fairly recent member of the B-complex family.

Usually measured in micrograms (mcg.).

Synthesis of ascorbic acid requires biotin.

Essential for normal metabolism of fat and protein.

The RDA for adults is 150 to 300 mcg.

Can be synthesized by intestinal bacteria.

Raw eggs prevent absorption by the body.

Synergistic with B_2, B_6, niacin, A, and in maintaining healthy skin.

WHAT IT CAN DO FOR YOU:

Aid in keeping hair from turning gray.

Help in preventive treatment for baldness.

Ease muscle pains.

Alleviate eczema and dermatitis.

DEFICIENCY DISEASE:

Eczema of face and body, extreme exhaustion, impairment of fat metabolism. (For deficiency symptoms, see section 76.)

BEST NATURAL SOURCES:

Nuts, fruits, brewer's yeast, beef liver, egg yolk, milk, kidney, and unpolished rice.

SUPPLEMENTS:

Biotin is usually included in most B-complex supplements and multiple-vitamin tablets.

Daily doses most often used are 25 to 300 mcg.

TOXICITY:

There are no known cases of biotin toxicity.

ENEMIES:

Raw egg white (which contains avidin, a protein that prevents biotin absorption), water, sulfa drugs, estrogen, food-processing techniques, and alcohol. (See section 206.)

PERSONAL ADVICE:

If you drink a lot of eggnogs made with raw eggs you probably need biotin supplementation.

Be sure you're getting at least 25 mcg. daily if you are on antibiotics or sulfa drugs.

Balding men might find that a biotin supplement may keep their hair there longer.

33. Vitamin C (Ascorbic Acid, Cevitamin Acid)

FACTS:

Water soluble.

Most animals synthesize their own vitamin C, but man, apes, and guinea pigs must rely upon dietary sources.

Plays a primary role in the formation of collagen, which is important for the growth and repair of body tissue cells, gums, blood vessels, bones, and teeth.

Helps in the body's absorption of iron.

Measured in milligrams (mg.).

Used up more rapidly under stress conditions.

The RDA for adults is 45 mg. (higher doses recommended during pregnancy and lactation).

Recommended as a preventive for crib death or sudden infant death syndrome (SIDS).

Smokers and older persons have greater need for vitamin C. (Each cigarette destroys 25 mg.)

WHAT IT CAN DO FOR YOU:

Heal wounds, burns, and bleeding gums.

Accelerate healing after surgery.

Help in decreasing blood cholesterol.

Aid in preventing many types of viral and bacterial infections.

Act as a natural laxative.

Lower incidence of blood clots in veins.

Aid in treatment and prevention of the common cold.

Extend life by enabling protein cells to hold together.

Reduce effects of many allergy-producing substances.

Prevent scurvy.

Decrease infections by 25 percent and cancers by 75 percent if taken in 1,000-mg. to 10,000-mg. daily dosage, according to Dr. Linus Pauling.

DEFICIENCY DISEASE:

Scurvy. (For deficiency symptoms, see section 76.)

BEST NATURAL SOURCES:

Citrus fruits, berries, green and leafy vegetables, tomatoes, cauliflower, potatoes, and sweet potatoes.

SUPPLEMENTS:

Vitamin C is one of the most widely taken supplements. It is available in conventional pills, time-release tablets, syrups, powders, chewable wafers, in just about every form a vitamin can take.

The form that is *pure* vitamin C is derived from corn dextrose (though no corn or dextrose remains).

The difference between "natural" or "organic" vitamin C and ordinary ascorbic acid is primarily in the individual's ability to digest it.

The best vitamin-C supplement is one that contains the complete C complex of bioflavonoids, hesperidin, and rutin. (Sometimes these are labeled citrus salts.)

Tablets and capsules are usually supplied in strengths up to 1,000 mg., and in powder form sometimes 5,000 mg. per tsp.

Daily doses most often used are 500 mg. to 4 g.

Rose hips vitamin C contains bioflavonoids and other enzymes that help C assimilate. They are the richest natural source of vitamin C. (The C is actually manufactured under the bud of the rose—called a hip.)

Acerola C is made with acerola berries.

TOXICITY:

No proven toxic effects, though excessive intake might cause some unpleasant side effects in specific cases. Occasional diarrhea, excess urination, kidney stones, and skin rashes may develop on megadoses. Cut back dosage if any of these occurs.

ENEMIES:

Water, cooking, heat, light, oxygen, smoking. (See section 206.)

PERSONAL ADVICE:

Because vitamin C is excreted in two to three hours, depending on the quantity of food in the stomach, and it is important to maintain a constant high level of C in the bloodstream at all times, I recommend a time-release tablet for optimal effectiveness.

If you're taking over 750 mg. daily, I suggest a magnesium supplement. This is an effective deterrent against kidney stones.

Carbon monoxide destroys vitamin C, so city dwellers should definitely up their intake.

You need extra C if you are on the pill.

I recommend increasing C doses if you take aspirin or simply want your other vitamins to work better.

If you take ginseng, it's better to take it three hours before or after taking vitamin C or foods high in the vitamin.

34. Calcium Pantothenate (Pantothenic Acid, Panthenol, Vitamin B₅)

FACTS:

Water soluble, another member of the B-complex family.

Helps in cell building, maintaining normal growth, and development of the central nervous system.

Vital for the proper functioning of the adrenal glands.

Essential for conversion of fat and sugar to energy.

Necessary for synthesis of antibodies, for utilization of PABA and choline.

The RDA (as set by the FDA) is 10 mg. for adults.

Can be synthesized in the body by intestinal bacteria.

WHAT IT CAN DO FOR YOU:

Aid in wound healing.
Fight infection by building antibodies.
Treat postoperative shock.

Prevent fatigue.

Reduce adverse and toxic effects of many antibiotics.

DEFICIENCY DISEASE:

Hypoglycemia, duodenal ulcers, blood and skin disorders. (For deficiency symptoms, see section 76.)

BEST NATURAL SOURCES:

Meat, whole grains, wheat germ, bran, kidney, liver, heart, green vegetables, brewer's yeast, nuts, chicken, crude molasses.

SUPPLEMENTS:

Most commonly found in B-complex formulas in a variety of strengths from 10 to 100 mg.

10 to 300 mg. are the daily doses usually taken.

TOXICITY:

No known toxic effects.

ENEMIES:

Heat, food-processing techniques, canning, caffeine, sulfa drugs, sleeping pills, estrogen, alcohol. (See section 206.)

PERSONAL ADVICE:

If you frequently have tingling hands and feet, you might try increasing your pantothenic acid intake—in combination with other B vitamins.

Pantothenic acid can help provide a defense against a stress situation that you foresee or are involved in.

1,000 mg. daily has been found effective in reducing the pain of arthritis, in some cases.

35. Choline

FACTS:

A member of the B-complex family and a lipotropic (fat emulsifier).

Works with inositol (another B-complex member) to utilize fats and cholesterol.

One of the few substances able to penetrate the so-called blood-brain barrier, which ordinarily protects the brain against variations in the daily diet, and go directly into the brain cells to produce a chemical that aids memory.

The RDA has not yet been established, though it's estimated that the average adult diet contains between 500 and 900 mg. a day.

Seems to emulsify cholesterol so that it doesn't settle on artery walls or in the gallbladder.

WHAT IT CAN DO FOR YOU:

Help control cholesterol buildup.

Aid in the sending of nerve impulses, specifically those in the brain used in the formation of memory.

Assist in conquering the problem of memory loss in later years.

Help eliminate poisons and drugs from your system by aiding the liver.

Produce a soothing effect.

DEFICIENCY DISEASE:

May result in cirrhosis and fatty degeneration of liver, hardening of the arteries, and possibly Alzheimer's disease. (For deficiency symptoms, see section 76.)

BEST NATURAL SOURCES:

Egg yolks, brain, heart, green leafy vegetables, yeast, liver, wheat germ, and, in small amounts, in lecithin.

SUPPLEMENTS:

Six lecithin capsules, made from soybeans, contain 244 mg. each of inositol and choline.

The average B-complex supplement contains approximately 50 mg. of choline and inositol.

Daily doses most often used are 500 to 1,000 mg.

TOXICITY:

None known.

ENEMIES:

Water, sulfa drugs, estrogen, food processing, and alcohol. (See section 206.)

PERSONAL ADVICE:

Always take choline with your other B vitamins.

If you are often nervous or "twitchy" it might help to increase your choline.

If you are taking lecithin, you probably need a chelated calcium supplement to keep your phosphorus and calcium in balance, since choline seems to increase the body's phosphorus.

Try getting more choline into your diet as a way to a better memory.

36. Vitamin D (Calciferol, Viosterol, Ergosterol, "Sunshine Vitamin")

FACTS:

Fat soluble. Acquired through sunlight or diet. (Ultraviolet sunrays act on the oils of the skin to produce the vitamin, which is then absorbed into the body.)

When taken orally, vitamin D is absorbed with fats through the intestinal walls.

Measured in International Units (IU).

The RDA for adults is 400 IU.

Smog reduces the vitamin-D–producing sunshine rays.

After a suntan is established, vitamin-D production through the skin stops.

WHAT IT CAN DO FOR YOU:

Properly utilize calcium and phosphorus necessary for strong bones and teeth.

Taken with vitamins A and C it can aid in preventing colds.

Help in treatment of conjunctivitis.

Aid in assimilating vitamin A.

DEFICIENCY DISEASE:

Rickets, severe tooth decay, osteomalacia, senile osteoporis. (For deficiency symptoms, see section 76.)

Best Natural Sources:

Fish liver oils, sardines, herring, salmon, tuna, milk and dairy products.

Supplements:

Usually supplied in 400 IU capsules, the vitamin itself is derived from fish liver oil.

Daily doses most often taken are 400 to 1,000 IU.

Toxicity:

25,000 IU daily over an extended period of time can produce toxic effects in adults.

Dosages of over 5,000 IU daily might affect some individuals adversely.

Signs of toxicity are unusual thirst, sore eyes, itching skin, vomiting, diarrhea, urinary urgency, abnormal calcium deposits in blood-vessel walls, liver, lungs, kidney, and stomach.

Enemies:

Mineral oil, smog. (See section 206.)

Personal Advice:

City dwellers, especially those in areas of high smog density, should increase their vitamin-D intake.

Night workers, nuns, and others whose clothing or life-style keeps them from sunlight should increase the D in their diet.

Children who don't drink D-fortified milk should increase their intake of D.

Dark-skinned people living in northern climates usually need an increase in vitamin D.

Do not supplement your dog's or cat's diet with vitamin D unless your vet specifically advises it. (See section 98.)

37. Vitamin E (Tocopherol)

FACTS:

Fat soluble and stored in the liver, fatty tissues, heart, muscles, testes, uterus, blood, adrenal and pituitary glands.

Formerly measured by weight, but now generally designated according to its biological activity in International Units (IU). With this vitamin 1 IU is the same as 1 mg.

Composed of compounds called tocopherols. Of the eight tocopherols—alpha, beta, gamma, delta, epsilon, zeta, eta, and theta—alphatocopherol is the most effective.

An active antioxidant, prevents oxidation of fat compounds as well as that of vitamin A, selenium, two sulfur amino acids, and some vitamin C.

Enhances activity of vitamin A.

The RDA for adults is 12 IU to 15 IU. (This requirement is based on the National Research Council's 1974 revised allowances. The U.S. RDA for adults is 30 IU.)

60 to 70 percent of daily doses are excreted in feces. Unlike other fat-soluble vitamins, E is stored in the body for a relatively short time, much like B and C.

Important as a vasodilator and an anticoagulant.

Products with 25 mcg. of selenium for each 200 units of E increase E's potency.

WHAT IT CAN DO FOR YOU:

Keep you looking younger by retarding cellular aging due to oxidation.

Supply oxygen to the body to give you more endurance.

Protect your lungs against air pollution by working with vitamin A.

Prevent and dissolve blood clots.

Alleviate fatigue.

Prevent thick scar formation externally (when applied topically—it can be absorbed through the skin) and internally.

Accelerate healing of burns.

Working as a diuretic, it can lower blood pressure.

Aid in prevention of miscarriages.

DEFICIENCY DISEASE:

Destruction of red blood cells, muscle degeneration, some anemias and reproductive disorders. (For deficiency symptoms, see section 76.)

BEST NATURAL SOURCES:

Wheat germ, soybeans, vegetable oils, broccoli, Brussels sprouts, leafy greens, spinach, enriched flour, whole wheat, whole-grain cereals, and eggs.

SUPPLEMENTS:

Available in oil-base capsules as well as water-soluble dry-base tablets.

Usually supplied in strengths from 100 to 1,000 IU. The dry form is recommended for anyone who cannot tolerate oil or whose skin condition is aggravated by oil.

Daily doses most often used are 200 to 1,200 IU.

TOXICITY:

Essentially nontoxic.

ENEMIES:

Heat, oxygen, freezing temperatures, food processing, iron, chlorine, mineral oil. (See section 206.)

PERSONAL ADVICE:

If you're on a diet high in polyunsaturated oils, you might need additional vitamin E.

Inorganic iron (ferrous sulfate) destroys vitamin E, so the two should not be taken together. If you're using a supplement containing any ferrous sulfate, E should be taken at least eight hours before or after.

Ferrous gluconate, peptonate, citrate, or fumerate (organic iron complexes) do not destroy E.

If you have chlorinated drinking water, you need more vitamin E.

Pregnant or lactating women, as well as those on the pill or taking hormones, need increased vitamin E.

I advise women going through menopause to increase their E intake.

38. Vitamin F (Unsaturated Fatty Acids—Linoleic, and Arachidonic)

FACTS:

Fat soluble, made up of unsaturated fatty acids obtained from foods.

Measured in milligrams (mg.).

No RDA has been established, but the National Research Council has suggested that at least 1 percent of total calories should include essential unsaturated fatty acids.

Unsaturated fat helps burn saturated fat, with intake balanced two to one.

Twelve teaspoons sunflower seeds or eighteen pecan halves can furnish a day's complete supply.

If there is sufficient linoleic acid, the other two fatty acids can be synthesized.

Heavy carbohydrate consumption increases need.

WHAT IT CAN DO FOR YOU:

Aid in preventing cholesterol deposits in the arteries.

Promote healthy skin and hair.

Give some degree of protection against the harmful effects of X-rays.

Aid in growth and well-being by influencing glandular activity and making calcium available to cells.

Combat heart disease.

Aid in weight reduction by burning saturated fats.

Deficiency Disease:

Eczema, acne. (For deficiency symptoms, see section 76.)

Best Natural Sources:

Vegetable oils—wheat germ, linseed, sunflower, safflower, soybean, and peanut—peanuts, sunflower seeds, walnuts, pecans, almonds, avocados.

Supplements:

Comes in capsules of 100- to 150-mg. strengths.

Toxicity:

No known toxic effects, but an excess can lead to unwanted pounds.

Enemies:

Saturated fats, heat, oxygen.

Personal Advice:

For best absorption of vitamin F, take vitamin E with it at mealtimes.

If you are a heavy carbohydrate consumer, you need more vitamin F.

Anyone worried about cholesterol buildup should be getting the proper intake of F.

Though most nuts are fine sources of unsaturated fatty acids, Brazil nuts and cashews are *not*.

Watch out for fad diets high in saturated fats.

39. Folic Acid (Folacin)

FACTS:

Water soluble, another member of the B complex.

Measured in micrograms (mcg.).

Essential to the formation of red blood cells.

Aid in protein metabolism.

The official Recommended Daily Dietary Allowance for adults is 400 mcg., and twice that amount for pregnant and lactating women.

Important for the production of nucleic acids (RNA and DNA).

Essential for division of body cells.

Needed for utilization of sugar and amino acids.

Can be destroyed by being stored, unprotected, at room temperature for extended time periods.

WHAT IT CAN DO FOR YOU:

Improve lactation.

Protect against intestinal parasites and food poisoning.

Promote healthier-looking skin.

Act as an analgesic for pain.

May delay hair graying when used in conjunction with pantothenic acid and PABA.

Increase appetite, if you are debilitated (run down).

Act as a preventive for canker sores.
Help ward off anemia.

DEFICIENCY DISEASE:

Nutritional macrocytic anemia. (For deficiency symptoms, see section 76.)

BEST NATURAL SOURCES:

Deep-green leafy vegetables, carrots, tortula yeast, liver, egg yolk, cantaloupe, apricots, pumpkins, avocados, beans, whole wheat and dark rye flour.

SUPPLEMENTS:

Usually supplied in 400-mcg. and 800-mcg. strengths. Strengths of 1 mg. (1,000 mcg.) are available by prescription only.

400 mcg. are sometimes supplied in B-complex formulas, but often only 100 mcg. (Check labels.)

Daily doses most often used are 400 mcg. to 5 mg.

TOXICITY:

No known toxic effects, though a few people experience allergic skin reactions.

ENEMIES:

Water, sulfa drugs, sunlight, estrogen, food processing (especially boiling), heat. (See section 206.)

If you are a heavy drinker, it is advisable to increase your folic-acid intake.

High vitamin-C intake increases excretion of folic acid, and anyone taking more than 2 g. of C should probably up his folic acid.

If you are on Dilantin or take estrogens, sulfonamides, phenobarbital, or aspirin, I suggest increasing folic acid.

I've found that many people taking 1 to 5 mg. daily, for a short period of time, have reversed several types of skin discoloration. If this is a problem to you, it's worth checking out a nutritionally oriented doctor about the possibility.

If you are getting sick, or fighting an illness, make sure your stress supplement has ample folic acid. When folic acid is deficient, so are your antibodies.

40. Inositol

FACTS:

Water soluble, another member of the B complex, and a lipotropic.

Measured in milligrams (mg.).

Combines with choline to form lecithin.

Metabolizes fats and cholesterol.

Daily dietary allowances have not yet been established, but the average healthy adult gets approximately 1 g. a day.

Like choline, it has been found important in nourishing brain cells.

What It Can Do For You:

Help lower cholesterol levels.

Promote healthy hair—aid in preventing fall-out.

Help in preventing eczema.

Aid in redistribution of body fat.

Deficiency Disease:

Eczema. (For deficiency symptoms, see section 76.)

Best Natural Sources:

Liver, brewer's yeast, dried lima beans, beef brains and heart, cantaloupe, grapefruit, raisins, wheat germ, unrefined molasses, peanuts, cabbage.

Supplements:

As with choline, six soybean-based lecithin capsules contain approximately 244 mg. each of inositol and choline.

Available in lecithin powders that mix well with liquids. Most B-complex supplements contain approximately 100 mg. of choline and inositol.

Daily doses most often used are 250 to 500 mg.

Toxicity:

No known toxic effects.

Water, sulfa drugs, estrogen, food processing, alcohol, and coffee. (See section 206.)

PERSONAL ADVICE:

Take inositol with choline and your other B vitamins.

If you are a heavy coffee drinker, you probably need supplemental inositol.

If you take lecithin, I advise a supplement of chelated calcium to keep your phosphorus and calcium in balance, as both inositol and choline seem to raise phosphorus levels.

A good way to maximize the effectiveness of your vitamin E is to get enough inositol and choline.

41. Vitamin K (Menadione)

FACTS:

Fat soluble.

Usually measured in micrograms (mcg.).

There is a trio of K vitamins. K_1 and K_2 can be formed by natural bacteria in the intestines. K_3 is a synthetic.

No dietary allowance has yet been established, but an adult intake of approximately 300 mcg. is generally considered adequate. Newborn infants need more.

Essential in the formation of prothrombin, a blood-clotting chemical.

WHAT IT CAN DO FOR YOU:

Help in preventing internal bleeding and hemorrhages.

Aid in reducing excessive menstrual flow.
Promote proper blood clotting.

DEFICIENCY DISEASE:

Celiac disease, sprue, colitis. (For deficiency symptoms, see section 76.)

BEST NATURAL SOURCES:

Yogurt, alfalfa, egg yolk, safflower oil, soybean oil, fish liver oils, kelp, leafy green vegetables.

SUPPLEMENTS:

The abundance of natural vitamin K generally makes supplementation unnecessary.
Is is not included ordinarily in multiple-vitamin capsules.

TOXICITY:

More than 500 mcg. of synthetic vitamin K is not recommended.

ENEMIES:

X-rays and radiation, frozen foods, aspirin, air pollution, mineral oil. (See section 206.)

PERSONAL ADVICE:

Excessive diarrhea can be a symptom of vitamin-K deficiency, but before self-supplementing, see a doctor.

Yogurt is your best defense against a vita-min-K deficiency.

If you have nosebleeds often, try increasing your K through natural food sources. Alfalfa tablets might help.

42. Niacin (Nicotinic Acid, Niacinamide Nicotinamide)

FACTS:

Water soluble and a member of the B-complex family, known as B_3.

Usually measured in milligrams (mg).

Using the amino acid tryptophan, the body can manufacture its own niacin.

A person whose body is deficient in B_1, B_2, and B_6 will not be able to produce niacin from tryptophan.

Lack of niacin can bring about negative personality changes.

The RDA, according to the National Research Council, is 12 to 18 mg. for adults.

Essential for synthesis of sex hormones (estrogen, progestrone, testosterone), as well as cortisone, thyroxine, and insulin.

Necessary for healthy nervous system and brain function.

Niacinamide is more generally used since it minimizes the flushing and itching of the skin that frequently occurs with the nicotinic acid form of niacin. (The flush, by the way, is not serious and usually disappears in about twenty minutes.)

What It Can Do For You:

Aid in promoting a healthy digestive system, alleviate gastrointestinal disturbances.

Give you healthier-looking skin.

Help prevent and ease severity of migraine headaches.

Increase circulation and reduce high blood pressure.

Ease some attacks of diarrhea.

Reduce the unpleasant symptoms of vertigo in Ménière's syndrome.

Increase energy through proper utilization of food.

Help eliminate canker sores and, often, bad breath.

Reduce cholesterol.

Deficiency Disease:

Pellegra. (For deficiency symptoms, see setion 76.)

Best Natural Sources:

Liver, lean meat, whole wheat products, brewer's yeast, kidney, wheat germ, fish, eggs, roasted peanuts, the white meat of poultry, avocados, dates, figs, prunes.

Supplements:

Available as niacin and niacinamide. (The only difference is that niacin—nicotinic acid—might cause flushing and niacinamide—nicotinamide—will not. If you prefer niacin, you can minimize the flushing by taking your pill on a full stomach or with an equivalent amount of inositol.)

Usually found in 50- to 1,000-mg. doses in pill and powder form.

50 to 100 mg. are ordinarily included in the better B-complex formulas and multivitamin preparations. (Check labels.)

TOXICITY:

Essentially nontoxic, except for side effects resulting from doses above 100 mg.

Some sensitive individuals might evidence burning or itching skin.

Do not give to animals, especially dogs. (See section 98.)

ENEMIES:

Water, sulfa drugs, alcohol, food-processing techniques, sleeping pills, estrogen. (See section 206.)

PERSONAL ADVICE:

If you're taking antibiotics and suddenly find your niacin flushes becoming severe, don't be alarmed.

It's quite common. You'll probably be more comfortable if you switch to niacinamide.

If you have a cholesterol problem, increasing your niacin intake can help.

Skin that is particularly sensitive to sunlight is often an early indicator of niacin deficiency.

Do not give your pets large doses of niacin.

It can cause flushing and sweating, greatly distressing the animal and you.

43. Vitamin P (C Complex, Citrus Bioflavonoids, Rutin, Hesperidin)

FACTS:

Water soluble and composed of citrin, rutin, and hesperidin, as well as flavones and flavonals.

Usually measured in milligrams (mg.).

Necessary for the proper function and absorption of vitamin C.

Flavonoids are the substances that provide that yellow and orange color in citrus foods.

Also called the capillary permeability factor. (P stands for permeability.) The prime function of bioflavonoids is to increase capillary strength and regulate absorption.

Aids vitamin C in keeping connective tissues healthy.

No daily allowance has been established, but most nutritionists agree that for every 500 mg. of vitamin C you should have at least 100 mg. of bioflavonoids.

Works synergistically with vitamin C.

WHAT IT CAN DO FOR YOU:

Prevent vitamin C from being destroyed by oxidation.

Strengthen the walls of capillaries, thereby preventing bruising.

Help build resistance to infection.

Aid in preventing and healing bleeding gums.

Increase the effectiveness of vitamin C.

Help in the treatment of edema and dizziness due to disease of the inner ear.

DEFICIENCY DISEASE:

Capillary fragility. (For deficiency symptoms, see section 76.)

BEST NATURAL SOURCES:

The white skin and segment part of citrus fruit—lemons, oranges, grapefruit. Also in apricots, buckwheat, blackberries, cherries, and rose hips.

SUPPLEMENTS:

Available usually in a C complex or by itself. Most often there are 500 mg. of bioflavonoids to 50 mg. of rutin and hesperidin. (If the ratio of rutin and hesperidin is not equal, it should be twice as much rutin.)

All C supplements work better with bioflavonoids.

Most common doses of rutin and hesperidin are 100 mg. three times a day.

TOXICITY:

No known toxicity.

ENEMIES:

Menopausal women can usually find some effective relief from hot flashes with an increase in bioflavonoids taken in conjunction with vitamin C.

If your gums bleed frequently when you brush your teeth, make sure you're getting enough rutin and hesperidin.

Anyone with a tendency to bruise easily will benefit from a C supplement with bioflavonoids, rutin, and hesperidin.

44. PABA (Para-aminobenzoic Acid)

FACTS:

Water soluble, one of the newer members of the B-complex family.

Usually measured in milligrams (mg.).

Can be synthesized in the body.

No RDA has yet been established.

Helps form folic acid and is important in the utilization of protein.

Has important sun-screening properties.

Helps in the assimilation—and therefore the effectiveness—of pantothenic acid.

In experiments with animals, it has worked with pantothenic acid to restore gray hair to its natural color.

WHAT IT CAN DO FOR YOU:

Used as an ointment it can protect against sunburn.

Reduce the pain of burns.

Keep skin healthy and smooth.

Help in delaying wrinkles.

Help to restore natural color to your hair.

DEFICIENCY DISEASE:

Eczema. (For deficiency symptoms, see section 76.)

BEST NATURAL SOURCES:

Liver, brewer's yeast, kidney, whole grains, rice, bran, wheat germ, and molasses.

SUPPLEMENTS:

30 to 100 mg. are often included in good B-complex capsules as well as high-quality multivitamins.

Available in 30- to 1,000-mg. strengths in regular and time-release form.

Doses most often used are 30 to 100 mg. three times a day.

TOXICITY:

No known toxic effects, but long-term programs of high dosages are not recommended.

Symptoms that might indicate an oversupply of PABA are usually nausea and vomiting.

ENEMIES:

Water, sulfa drugs, food-processing techniques, alcohol, estrogen. (See section 206.)

PERSONAL ADVICE:

Some people claim that the combination of folic acid and PABA has returned their graying hair to its natural color. It has worked on animals, so it is certainly worth a try for anyone looking for an alternative to hair dye. For this purpose, 1,000 mg. (time release) daily for six days a week is a viable regimen.

If you tend to burn easily in the sun, use PABA as a protective ointment.

Many Hollywood celebrities I know use PABA to prevent wrinkles. It doesn't eliminate them, but it certainly seems to keep them at bay for some people.

If you are taking penicillin, or any sulfa drug, your PABA intake should be increased through natural foods or supplements.

45. Vitamin T

There is very little known about this vitamin, except that it helps in blood coagulation and the forming of platelets. Because of these attributes it is important in warding off certain forms of anemia and hemophilia. No RDA has been established, and there are no supplements for the public on the market. It is found in sesame seeds and egg yolks, and there is no known toxicity.

46. Vitamin U

Even less is known about vitamin U than vitamin T. It is reputed to play an important role in healing ulcers, but medical opinions vary on this. It is found in raw cabbage and no known toxicity exists.

IV

Your Mineral Essentials

47. Calcium

FACTS:

There is more calcium in the body than any other mineral.

Calcium and phosphorus work together for healthy bones and teeth.

Calcium and magnesium work together for cardiovascular health.

Almost all of the body's calcium (two to three pounds) is found in the bones and teeth.

20 percent of an adult's bone calcium is re-absorbed and replaced every year. (New bone cells form as old ones break down.)

Calcium must exist in a two-to-one relationship with phosphorus.

In order for calcium to be absorbed, the body must have sufficient vitamin D.

For adults, 800 to 1,200 mg. is the RDA.

Calcium and iron are the two minerals most deficient in the American woman's diet.

WHAT IT CAN DO FOR YOU:

Maintain strong bones and healthy teeth.
Keep your heart beating regularly.
Alleviate insomnia.
Help metabolize your body's iron.
Aid your nervous system, especially in impulse transmission.

DEFICIENCY DISEASE:

Rickets, osteomalacia, osteoporosis. (See section 76 for symptoms.)

BEST NATURAL SOURCES:

Milk and milk products, all cheeses, soybeans, sardines, salmon, peanuts, walnuts, sunflower seeds, dried beans, green vegetables.

SUPPLEMENTS:

Most often available in 100- to 500-mg. tablets.

Bonemeal is a fairly common supplement, and a good source of the mineral, though some people find calcium gluconate (a vegetarian source) or calcium lactate (a milk sugar derivative) easier to absorb. (Gluconate is more potent than lactate.)

The best form is chelated calcium tablets.

Many good multivitamin and mineral preparations include calcium.

When combined with magnesium, the ratio should be twice as much calcium as magnesium. Dolomite is a natural form of calcium and magnesium, and no vitamin D is needed for assimilation. Five dolomite tablets are equivalent to 750 mg. of calcium.

Doses most often used are 800 to 2,000 mg. per day.

TOXICITY:

Excessive daily intake of over 2,000 mg. might lead to hypercalcemia. (See section 98, "Cautions.")

ENEMIES:

Large quantities of fat, oxalic acid (found in chocolate and rhubarb), and phytic acid (found in grains) are capable of preventing proper calcium absorption.

PERSONAL ADVICE:

If you are afflicted with backaches, dolomite, chelated calcium, or bonemeal supplements might help.

Menstrual-cramp sufferers can often find relief by increasing their calcium intake.

Teenagers who suffer from "growing pains" will usually find that they disappear with an increase in calcium consumption.

Hypoglycemics could use more calcium.

48. Chlorine

FACTS:

Regulates the blood's alkaline–acid balance.
Works with sodium and potassium in a compound form.
Aids in the cleaning of body wastes by helping the liver to function.
No dietary allowance has been established, but if your daily salt intake is average, you are getting enough.

WHAT IT CAN DO FOR YOU:

Aid in digestion.
Help keep you limber.

DEFICIENCY DISEASE:

Loss of hair and teeth.

BEST NATURAL SOURCES:

Table salt, kelp, olives.

SUPPLEMENTS:

Most good multimineral preparations include it.

TOXICITY:

Over 15 g. can cause unpleasant side effects.

If you have chlorine in your drinking water, you aren't getting all the vitamin E you think. (Chlorinated water destroys vitamin E.)

Anyone who drinks chlorinated water would be well advised to eat yogurt—a good way to replace the intestinal bacteria the chlorine destroys.

49. Chromium

FACTS:

Works with insulin in the metabolism of sugar.

Helps bring protein to where it's needed.

No official dietary allowance has been established, but 90 mcg. is an average adult intake.

As you get older, you retain less chromium in your body.

WHAT IT CAN DO FOR YOU:

Aid growth.

Help prevent and lower high blood pressure.

Work as a deterrent for diabetes.

DEFICIENCY DISEASE:

A suspected factor in arteriosclerosis and diabetes.

BEST NATURAL SOURCES:

Meat, shellfish, chicken, corn oil, clams, brewer's yeast.

96

May be found in the better multimineral preparations.

TOXICITY:

No known toxicity.

PERSONAL ADVICE:

If you are low in chromium (a hair analysis can show this—see section 75), you might try a zinc supplement. For some reason, chelated zinc seems to substitute well for deficient chromium.

50. Cobalt

FACTS:

A mineral that is part of vitamin B_{12}.
Usually measured in micrograms (mcg.).
Essential for red blood cells.
Must be obtained from food sources.
No daily allowance has been set for this mineral, and only very small amounts are necessary in the diet (usually no more than 8 mcg.).

WHAT IT CAN DO FOR YOU:

Stave off anemia.

DEFICIENCY DISEASE:

Anemia.

BEST NATURAL SOURCES:

Meat, kidney, liver, milk, oysters, clams.

Rarely found in supplement form.

No known toxicity.

Whatever is antagonistic to B$_{12}$.

If you're a strict vegetarian, you are much more likely to be deficient in this mineral than someone who includes meat and shellfish in his or her diet.

51. Copper

Required to convert the body's iron into hemoglobin.

Can reach the bloodstream fifteen minutes after ingestion.

Makes the amino acid tyrosine usable, allowing it to work as the pigmenting factor for hair and skin.

Present in cigarettes, birth-control pills, and automobile pollution.

Essential for the utilization of vitamin C.

The RDA has not been set by the National Research Council, but 2 mg. for adults is suggested.

What It Can Do For You:

Keep your energy up by aiding in effective iron absorption.

Deficiency Disease:

Anemia, edema.

Best Natural Sources:

Dried beans, peas, whole wheat, prunes, calf and beef liver, shrimp, and most seafood.

Supplements:

Usually available in multivitamin and mineral supplements in 2-mg. doses.

Toxicity:

Rare. (See section 98, "Cautions.")

Enemies:

Not easily destroyed.

Personal Advice:

As essential as copper is, I rarely suggest special supplementation. An excess seems to lower zinc level and produce insomnia, hair loss, irregular menses, and depression.

If you eat enough whole-grain products and fresh green leafy vegetables, as well as liver, you don't have to worry about your copper intake.

52. Fluorine

FACTS:

Part of the synthetic compound sodium fluoride (the type added to drinking water) and calcium fluoride (a natural substance).

Decreases chances of dental caries, though too much can discolor teeth.

No RDA has been established, but most people get about 1 mg. daily from fluoridated drinking water.

WHAT IT CAN DO FOR YOU:

Reduce tooth decay.
Strengthen bones.

DEFICIENCY DISEASE:

Tooth decay.

BEST NATURAL SOURCES:

Fluoridated drinking water, seafoods, and gelatin.

SUPPLEMENTS:

Not ordinarily found in multimineral supplements.

Available in prescription multivitamins for children in areas without fluoridated water.

TOXICITY:

20 to 80 mg. per day.

Aluminum salts of fluorine.

PERSONAL ADVICE:

Don't take additional fluoride unless it is prescribed by a physician or dentist.

53. Iodine (Iodide)

FACTS:

Two-thirds of the body's iodine is in the thyroid gland.

Since the thyroid gland controls metabolism, and iodine influences the thyroid, an undersupply of this mineral can result in slow mental reaction, weight gain, and lack of energy.

The RDA, as established by the National Research Council, is 80 to 150 mcg. for adults (1 mcg. per kilogram of body weight) and 125 to 150 mcg. for pregnant and lactating women respectively.

WHAT IT CAN DO FOR YOU:

Help you with dieting by burning excess fat.
Promote proper growth.
Give you more energy.
Improve mental alacrity.
Promote healthy hair, nails, skin, and teeth.

DEFICIENCY DISEASE:

Goiter, hypothyroidism.

BEST NATURAL SOURCES:

Kelp, vegetables grown in iodine-rich soil, onions, and all seafood.

SUPPLEMENTS:

Available in multimineral and high-potency vitamin supplements in doses of 0.15 mg.

Natural kelp is a good source of supplemental iodine.

TOXICITY:

No known toxicity from natural iodine, though iodine as a drug can be harmful if prescribed incorrectly. (See section 98, "Cautions.")

ENEMIES:

Food processing, nutrient-poor soil.

PERSONAL ADVICE:

Aside from kelp, and the iodine included in multimineral and vitamin preparations, I don't recommend additional supplements unless you're advised by a doctor to take them.

If you use salt and live in the Midwest, where iodine-poor soil is common, make sure the salt is iodized.

If you are inclined to eat excessive amounts of raw cabbage, you might *not* be getting the iodine you need, because there are elements in the cabbage that prevent proper utilization of the iodine. This being the case, you should consider a kelp supplement.

54. Iron

FACTS:

Essential and required for life, necessary for the production of hemoglobin (red blood corpuscles), myoglobin (red pigment in muscles), and certain enzymes.

Iron and calcium are the two major dietary deficiencies of American women.

Only about 8 percent of your total iron intake is absorbed and actually enters your bloodstream.

An average 150-pound adult has about 4 g. of iron in his or her body. Hemoglobin, which accounts for most of the iron, is recycled and reutilized as blood cells are replaced every 120 days. Iron bound to protein (ferretin) is stored in the body, as is tissue iron (present in myoglobin) in very small amounts.

The RDA, according to the National Research Council, is 10 to 18 mg. for adults, and 18 mg. for pregnant and lactating women.

In one month, women lose almost twice as much iron as men.

Copper, cobalt, manganese, and vitamin C are necessary to assimilate iron. Iron is necessary for proper metabolization of B vitamins.

WHAT IT CAN DO FOR YOU:

Aid growth.
Promote resistance to disease.
Prevent fatigue.
Cure and prevent iron-deficiency anemia.
Bring back good skin tone.

DEFICIENCY DISEASE:

Iron-deficiency anemia. (For deficiency symptoms, see section 76.)

BEST NATURAL SOURCES:

Pork liver, beef kidney, heart and liver, farina, raw clams, dried peaches, red meat, egg yolks, oysters, nuts, beans, asparagus, molasses, oatmeal.

SUPPLEMENTS:

The most assimilable form of iron is hydrolyzed-protein chelate, which means organic iron that has been processed for fastest assimilation. This form is nonconstipating and easy on sensitive systems.

Ferrous sulfate, inorganic iron, appears in many vitamin and mineral supplements and can destroy vitamin E (they should be taken at least eight hours apart). Check labels; many drugstore formulas contain ferrous sulfate.

Supplements with organic iron—ferrous gluconate, ferrous fumerate, ferrous citrate, or ferrous peptonate—do not neutralize vitamin E. They are available in a wide variety of doses, usually up to 320 mg.

TOXICITY:

Rare in healthy, normal individuals. Excessive doses, though, can be a hazard for children. (See section 98, "Cautions.")

ENEMIES:

Phosphoproteins in eggs and phytates in un-leavened whole wheat reduce iron availability to body.

PERSONAL ADVICE:

If you are a woman, I recommend an iron supplement. Check the label on your multivita-min or mineral preparation and see what you are already getting and guide yourself accord-ingly. (Remember, if the iron in your prepara-tion is ferrous sulfate, you're losing your vita-min E.)

Keep your iron supplements out of the reach of children.

Coffee drinkers, as well as tea drinkers, be aware that if you consume large quantities of either beverage you are most likely inhibiting your iron absorption.

55. Magnesium

FACTS:

Necessary for calcium and vitamin-C metab-olism, as well as that of phosphorus, sodium, and potassium.

Measured in milligrams (mg.).

Essential for effective nerve and muscle func-tioning.

Important for converting blood sugar into energy.

Known as the antistress mineral.

Alcoholics are usually deficient.

Adults need 300 to 400 mg. daily, slightly

more for pregnant and lactating women, according to the National Research Council.

The human body contains approximately 21 g. of magnesium.

WHAT IT CAN DO FOR YOU:

Aid in fighting depression.

Promote a healthier cardiovascular system and help prevent heart attacks.

Keep teeth healthier.

Help prevent calcium deposits, kidney and gallstones.

Bring relief from indigestion.

DEFICIENCY DISEASE:

(For deficiency symptoms, see section 76.)

BEST NATURAL SOURCES:

Figs, lemons, grapefruit, yellow corn, almonds, nuts, seeds, dark-green vegetables, apples.

SUPPLEMENTS:

Dolomite, which has magnesium and calcium in perfect balance (half as much magnesium as calcium), is a fine magnesium supplement.

Available in multivitamin and mineral preparations (best if they are chelated).

Can be purchased as magnesium oxide. 250-mg. strength equals 150 mg. per tablet.

Commonly available in 133.3-mg. strengths and taken four times a day.

Supplements of magnesium should not be

taken after meals, since the mineral does neutralize stomach acidity.

TOXICITY:

Large amounts, over an extended period of time, can be toxic if your calcium and phosphorus intakes are high. (See section 98, "Cautions.")

ENEMIES:

Diuretics, alcohol. (See section 206.)

PERSONAL ADVICE:

If you are a drinker, I suggest you increase your intake of magnesium.

Women who are on the pill or taking estrogen in any form would be well advised to take larger amounts of magnesium.

If you are a heavy consumer of nuts, seeds, and green vegetables, you probably get ample magnesium—as does anyone who lives in an area with hard water.

56. Manganese

FACTS:

Helps activate enzymes necessary for the body's proper use of biotin, B_1, and vitamin C.

Needed for normal bone structure.

Measured in milligrams (mg.).

Important in the formation of thyroxin, the principal hormone of the thyroid gland.

Necessary for the proper digestion and utilization of food.

No official daily allowance has been set, but 2.5 to 7 mg. is generally accepted to be the average adult requirement.

Important for reproduction and normal central nervous system function.

What It Can Do For You:

Help eliminate fatigue.
Aid in muscle reflexes.
Improve memory.
Reduce nervous irritability.

Deficiency Disease:

Ataxia.

Best Natural Sources:

Nuts, green leafy vegetables, peas, beets, egg yolks, whole-grain cereals.

Supplements:

Most often found in multivitamin and mineral combinations in dosages of 1 to 9 mg.

Toxicity:

Rare, except from industrial sources. (See section 98, "Cautions.")

Enemies:

Large intakes of calcium and phosphorus will inhibit absorption.

If you suffer from recurrent dizziness, you might try adding more manganese to your diet.

I advise absentminded people, or anyone with memory problems, to make sure they are getting enough of this mineral.

Heavy milk drinkers and meat eaters need increased manganese.

57. Molybdenum

FACTS:

Aids in carbohydrate and fat metabolism.

A vital part of the enzyme responsible for iron utilization.

No dietary allowance has been set, but the estimated daily intake of 45 to 500 mcg. has generally been accepted as the adequate human requirement.

WHAT IT CAN DO FOR YOU:

Help in preventing anemia.
Promote general well-being.

DEFICIENCY DISEASE:

None known.

BEST NATURAL SOURCES:

Dark-green leafy vegetables, whole grains, legumes.

SUPPLEMENTS:

Not ordinarily available.

Rare, but 5 to 10 parts per million has been considered toxic.

PERSONAL ADVICE:

As important as molybdenum is, there seems no need for supplementation unless all the food you consume comes from nutrient-deficient soil.

58. Phosphorus

FACTS:

Present in every cell in the body.

Vitamin D and calcium are essential to proper phosphorus functioning.

Calcium and phosphorus should be balanced two to one to work correctly (twice as much calcium as phosphorus).

Involved in virtually all physiological chemical reactions.

Necessary for normal bone and tooth structure.

Niacin cannot be assimilated without phosphorus.

Important for heart regularity.

Essential for normal kidney functioning.

Needed for the transference of nerve impulses.

The RDA is 800 to 1,200 mg. for adults, the higher levels for pregnant and lactating women.

WHAT IT CAN DO FOR YOU:

Aid in growth and body repair.

Provide energy and vigor by helping in the metabolization of fats and starches.

110

Lessen the pain of arthritis.
Promote healthy gums and teeth.

DEFICIENCY DISEASE:

Rickets, pyorrhea.

BEST NATURAL SOURCES:

Fish, poultry, meat, whole grains, eggs, nuts, seeds.

SUPPLEMENTS:

Bonemeal is a fine natural source of phosphorus. (Make sure vitamin D has been added to help assimilation.)

TOXICITY:

No known toxicity. (See section 98, "Cautions.")

ENEMIES:

Too much iron, aluminum, and magnesium can render phosphorus ineffective.

PERSONAL ADVICE:

When you get too much phosphorus, you throw off your mineral balance and decrease your calcium. Our diets are usually high in phosphorus—since it does occur in almost every natural food—and therefore calcium deficiencies are frequent. Be aware of this and adjust your diet accordingly.

If you're over forty, you should cut down on your weekly meat consumption and eat more leafy vegetables and drink milk. The reason for this is that after forty our kidneys don't help excrete excess phosphorus, and calcium is again depleted. Be on the lookout for foods preserved with phosphates and consider that as part of your phosphorus intake.

59. Potassium

FACTS:

Works with sodium to regulate the body's water balance and normalize heart rhythms. (Potassium works inside the cells, sodium works just outside them.)

Nerve and muscle functions suffer when the sodium–potassium balance is off.

Hypoglycemia (low blood sugar) causes potassium loss, as does a long fast or severe diarrhea.

No dietary allowance has been set, but approximately 900 mg. is considered a healthy daily intake.

Both mental and physical stress can lead to a potassium deficiency.

WHAT IT CAN DO FOR YOU:

Aid in clear thinking by sending oxygen to brain.

Help dispose of body wastes.

Assist in reducing blood pressure.

Aid in allergy treatment.

DEFICIENCY DISEASE:

Edema, hypoglycemia. (For deficiency symptoms, see section 76.)

Best Natural Sources:

Citrus fruits, watercress, all green leafy vegetables, mint leaves, sunflower seeds, bananas, potatoes.

Supplements:

Available in most high-potency multivitamin and multimineral preparations.

Inorganic potassium "salts" are the sulfate (alum), the chloride, the oxide, and carbonate. Organic potassium refers to the gluconate, the citrate, the fumerate.

Can be bought separately as potassium gluconate in dosages up to nearly 600 mg.

Toxicity:

25 g. of potassium chloride can cause toxicity. (See section 98, "Cautions.")

Enemies:

Alcohol, coffee, sugar, diuretics. (See section 206.)

Personal Advice:

If you drink large amounts of coffee, you might find that the fatigue you're fighting is due to the potassium loss you're suffering from.

Heavy drinkers and anyone wth a hungry sweet tooth should be aware that their potassium levels are probably low.

If you have low blood sugar, you are likely to be losing potassium while retaining water. And if you take a diuretic, you'll lose even more potassium! Watch your diet, increase your green vegetables, and take enough magnesium to regain your mineral balance.

Losing weight on a low-carbohydrate diet might not be the only thing you're losing. Chances are your potassium level is down. Watch out for weakness and poor reflexes.

60. Selenium

FACTS:

Vitamin E and selenium are synergistic. This means that the two together are stronger than the sum of the equal parts.

Both vitamin E and selenium are antioxidants, preventing or at least slowing down aging and hardening of tissues through oxidation.

Males appear to have a greater need for selenium. Almost half their body's supply concentrates in the testicles and portions of the seminal ducts adjacent to the prostate gland. Also, selenium is lost in the semen.

No official dietary allowance has yet been set for this mineral, but the general dosage is between 50 and 100 mcg. It is not advisable to exceed 200 mcg. daily.

WHAT IT CAN DO FOR YOU:

Aid in keeping youthful elasticity in tissues.

Alleviate hot flashes and menopausal distress.

Help in treatment and prevention of dandruff.

Possibly neutralize certain carcinogens and provide protection from some cancers.

DEFICIENCY DISEASE:

Premature stamina loss.

BEST NATURAL SOURCES:

Wheat germ, bran, tunafish, onions, tomatoes, broccoli.

SUPPLEMENTS:

Available in small microgram doses. 25 to 50 mcg. is most often used.

Also available combined with vitamin E and other antioxidants.

Natural foods supply sufficient amounts when eaten regularly.

TOXICITY:

Doses above 5 parts per million can be toxic.

ENEMIES:

Food-processing techniques.

PERSONAL ADVICE:

Selenium was discovered only a little more than twenty years ago. We've just begun to recognize its importance in human nutrition. Until more is known, I advise taking only moderate supplements.

61. Sodium

FACTS:

Sodium and potassium were discovered together and both found to be essential for normal growth.

High intakes of sodium (salt) will result in a depletion of potassium.

Diets high in sodium usually account for many instances of high blood pressure.

There is no official allowance, but a daily single gram of sodium chloride has been suggested for each kilogram of water drunk. Sodium aids in keeping calcium and other minerals in the blood soluble.

WHAT IT CAN DO FOR YOU:

Aid in preventing heat prostration or sunstroke.

Help your nerves and muscles function properly.

DEFICIENCY DISEASE:

Impaired carbohydrates digestion, possibly neuralgia.

BEST NATURAL SOURCES:

Salt, shellfish, carrots, beets, artichokes, dried beef, brains, kidney, bacon.

SUPPLEMENTS:

Rarely needed, but if so, kelp is a safe and nutritive supplement.

TOXICITY:

Over 14 g. of sodium chloride daily can produce toxic effects.

PERSONAL ADVICE:

If you think you don't eat much salt, see section 236 and think again.

If you have high blood pressure, cut down on your sodium intake by reading the labels on the foods you buy. Look for SALT, SODIUM, or the chemical symbol *Na*.

Adding sodium to your diet is as easy as a shake of salt, but subtracting it can be difficult. Avoid luncheon meats, frankfurters, salted cured meats such as ham, bacon, corned beef, as well as condiments—ketchup, chili sauce, soy sauce, mustard. Don't use baking powder or baking soda in cooking.

62. Sulfur

FACTS:

Essential for healthy hair, skin, and nails.

Helps maintain oxygen balance necessary for proper brain function.

Works with B-complex vitamins for basic body metabolism, and is part of tissue-building amino acids.

Aids the liver in bile secretion.

No RDA has been set, but a diet sufficient in protein will generally be sufficient in sulfur.

WHAT IT CAN DO FOR YOU:

Tone up skin and make hair more lustrous.

Help fight bacterial infections.

117

DEFICIENCY DISEASE:

None known.

BEST NATURAL SOURCES:

Lean beef, dried beans, fish, eggs, cabbage.

SUPPLEMENTS:

Not readily available as a food supplement.
Can be found in topical ointments and creams for skin problems.

TOXICITY:

No known toxicity from organic sulfur, but ill effects may occur from large amounts of inorganic sulfur.

PERSONAL ADVICE:

If you're getting enough protein in your daily meals, you are, most likely, getting enough sulfur.

Sulfur creams and ointments have been remarkably successful in treating a variety of skin problems. Check the ingredients in the preparation you are now using. There are many fine natural preparations available at health-food centers.

63. Vanadium

FACTS:

Inhibits the formation of cholesterol in blood vessels.

No dietary allowance set.

What It Can Do For You:

Aid in preventing heart attacks.

Deficiency Disease:

None known.

Best Natural Sources:

Fish.

Supplements:

Not available.

Toxicity:

Can easily be toxic if taken in synthetic form.

Personal Advice:

This is not one of the minerals that needs to be supplemented. A good fish dinner will supply you with the vanadium you need.

64. Zinc

Facts:

Zinc acts as a traffic policeman, directing and overseeing the efficient flow of body processes, the maintenance of enzyme systems and cells.

Essential for protein synthesis.

Governs the contractibility of muscles.

Helps in the formation of insulin.

Important for blood stability and in maintaining the body's acid-alkaline balance.

Exerts a normalizing effect on the prostate and is important in the development of all reproductive organs.

New studies indicate its importance in brain function and the treatment of schizophrenia.

Strong evidence of its requirement for the synthesis of DNA.

The RDA, as set by the National Research Council, is 15 mg. for adults (slightly higher allowances for pregnant and lactating women).

Excessive sweating can cause a loss of as much as 3 mg. of zinc per day.

Most zinc in foods is lost in processing, or never exists in substantial amount due to nutrient-poor soil.

WHAT IT CAN DO FOR YOU:

Accelerate healing time for internal and external wounds.

Get rid of white spots on the fingernails.

Help eliminate loss of taste.

Aid in the treatment of infertility.

Help avoid prostate problems.

Promote growth and mental alertness.

Help decrease cholesterol deposits.

DEFICIENCY DISEASE:

Possibly prostatic hypertrophy (noncancerous enlargement of the prostate gland), arteriosclerosis.

BEST NATURAL SOURCES:

Round steak, lamb chops, pork loin, wheat germ, brewer's yeast, pumpkin seeds, eggs, nonfat dry milk, ground mustard.

SUPPLEMENTS:

Available in all good multivitamin and multimineral preparations.

Can be bought as zinc-sulfate or zinc-gluconate tablets in doses ranging from 15 to over 300 mg. Both zinc sulfate and zinc gluconate seem to be equally effective, but zinc gluconate appears to be more easily tolerated.

Chelated zinc is the best way to take zinc.

Zinc is also available in combination with vitamin C, magnesium, and the B-complex vitamins.

TOXICITY:

Virtually nontoxic, except when there is an excessive intake and the food ingested has been stored in galvanized containers. Doses over 150 mg. are not recommended. (See section 98, "Cautions.")

PERSONAL ADVICE:

You need higher intakes of zinc if you are taking large amounts of vitamin B_6. This is also true if you are an alcoholic or a diabetic.

Men with prostate problems—and without them—would be well advised to keep their zinc levels up.

I have seen success in cases of impotence with a supplement program of B_6 and zinc.

Elderly people, concerned about senility, might find a zinc and manganese supplement beneficial.

If you are bothered by irregular menses, you might try a zinc supplement before resorting to hormone treatment to establish regularity.

Remember, if you are adding zinc to your diet, you will increase your need for vitamin A.

65. Water

FACTS:

The simple truth is that this is our most important nutrient. One-half to three-fourths of the body's weight is water.

A human being can live for weeks without food, but only a few days without water.

Water is the basic solvent for all the products of digestion.

Essential for removing wastes.

There is no specific dietary allowance since water loss varies with climate, situations, and individuals, but under ordinary circumstances six glasses daily is considered healthy.

Regulates body temperature.

WHAT IT CAN DO FOR YOU:

Keep all your bodily functions functioning.

Aid in dieting by depressing appetite before meals.

Help prevent constipation.

DEFICIENCY DISEASE:

Dehydration.

BEST NATURAL SOURCES:

Drinking water, juices, fruits, and vegetables.

SUPPLEMENTS:

All drinkable liquids can substitute for our daily water requirements.

TOXICITY:

No known toxicity, but an intake of one and a half gallons (that's sixteen to twenty-four glasses) in about an hour could be dangerous to an adult. It could kill an infant.

PERSONAL ADVICE:

I advise six to eight glasses of water daily, to be drunk a half hour before meals, for anyone who's dieting.

If you're running a fever, be sure to drink lots of water to prevent dehydration and to flush system of wastes.

If you live in an area where there is hard water, you're probably getting more calcium and magnesium than you think.

V

Other Wonder Workers

66. Acidophilus

Lactobacilus acidophilus, or acidophilus, as it is commonly known, is a source of friendly intestinal bacteria and more effective than yogurt. It is available as acidophilus culture, incubated in soy, milk, or yeast bases.

> Regular use of acidophilus keeps
> the intestines clean.

Many doctors prescribe acidophilus in conjunction with oral antibiotic treatment because antibiotics destroy beneficial intestinal flora, often causing diarrhea as well as an overgrowth of the fungus monilia abricans. This fungus can grow in the intestines, vagina, lungs, mouth (thrush), on the fingers, or under the nails. It will usually disappear after a few days use of generous amounts of acidophilus culture.

Regular use of acidophilus culture keeps the intestines clean. It can eliminate bad breath caused by intestinal putrefaction (the sort resistant to mouthwash or breath spray), constipation, foul-smelling flatulence, and aid in the treatment of acne and other skin problems.

Keep in mind that lactose, complex carbohydrates, pectin, and vitamin C plus roughage encourage additional growth of intestinal flora. This is important since friendly bacteria can die within five days unless they are continuously supplied with some form of lactic acid or lactose—like acidophilus.

67. Ginseng

It is generally well accepted that ginseng is a stimulant of both mental and physical energy. The Chinese have been using it for nearly five thousand years and still revere it as a preventive and cure-all. It is a mild laxative and helps the body pass poisons through more rapidly. Its reputed benefits include cures for impotence, high and low blood pressure, anemia, arthritis, indigestion, insomnia, fatigue, hypoglycemia, poor circulation, and more.

Miracles aside, ginseng does help you assimilate vitamins and minerals by acting as an endocrine-gland stimulant. It is best to take it on an empty stomach, preferably before breakfast, if you want it to be its most effective.

Vitamin C has been said to neutralize part of ginseng's value, but there is no real evidence to support this. (If you take a vitamin-C supplement, the time-release form makes any counteraction less likely.)

Ginseng is available in capsule form, under names such as Siberian ginseng and Korean ginseng, in 500-mg. to 650-mg. (10-grain) doses. It can also be purchased as tea, liquid concentrate, or as ginseng root in a bottle.

68. Alfalfa, Garlic, Chlorophyll, and Yucca

A natural diuretic

Alfalfa has been dubbed "the great healer" by noted biologist and author Frank Bouer, who discovered that the green leaves of this remarkable legume contain *eight* essential enzymes. Also, for every 100 g., it contains 8,000 IU of vitamin A and 20,000 to 40,000 units of vitamin K, which protects against hemorrhaging and helps in blood clotting. It is additionally a fine source of vitamins B₆ and E, and contains enough vitamin D, lime, and phosphorus to secure strong bones and teeth in growing children.

Many doctors have used alfalfa in treating stomach ailments, gas pains, ulcerous conditions, and poor appetite because it contains vitamin U, which is also found in raw cabbage and cabbage juice. The latter has frequently been used as an aid in treating peptic ulcers. Alfalfa is also a good laxative and a natural diuretic.

"Russian penicillin"

Garlic contains potassium, phosphorus, a significant amount of B and C vitamins, as well as calcium and protein. In Europe it is respected as a valuable medicine. The Soviets call it "Russian penicillin." In America it is virtually ignored.

Despite its small acceptance here, it does appear to have some amazing properties. Many medical authorities feel that it can reduce high blood pressure by either neutralizing the poisonous substances in the intestines or acting as a vasodilator. F. G. Piotrousky, of the University of Vienna, found that 40 percent of his hypertensive patients had substantially lower blood pressure after they were given garlic.

Garlic has also been found to be effective in cleansing the blood of excess glucose. (Blood sugar ranks with cholesterol as a causative factor in arteriosclerosis and heart attacks.) In addition, it has also been reported to alleviate grippe, sore throat, and bronchial congestion.

The best way to take garlic as a supplement is in the form of perles. These caps contain the valuable garlic oils and leave no after-odor on the breath, because they do not dissolve in the stomach but in the lower digestive tract. Garlic tablets with parsley (which contains natural chlorophyll) are also available.

Chlorophyll, according to G. W. Rapp in the *American Journal of Pharmacy,* possesses positive antibacterial action. It also appears to act as a wound-healing agent, and, while stimulating the growth of new tissue, it reduces the hazard of bacterial contamination.

Nature's deodorant, it is used in commercial air fresheners, as a topical body deodorant and as an oral breath refresher. It is available in tablets and in liquid preparations.

Yucca extract comes from the genus of trees and shrubs belonging to the Liliaceae family. (The Joshua tree is a yucca.) The Indians used the yucca for many purposes and revered it as a plant that guaranteed their health and survival. Dr. John W. Yale, a botanical biochemist, extracted the steroid saponin from the plant and used the extract in a tablet for the treatment of arthritis. The treatment proved safe and effective, the average dose being four tablets daily, and there was no gastrointestinal irritation. Yucca-extract tablets are nontoxic and available in most health-food and vitamin stores.

69. Bran and Fiber

Recent research appearing in the *Journal of the American Medical Association* indicates that we would all be a great deal healthier and live longer if we ate coarser diets that sent more indigestible dietary fiber through our digestive tracts.

CRUDE FIBER CONTENT OF THE U.S. DIET

1909	6.8 g./day
1957–59	4.9 g./day*
1979	about 4.9 g./day

*28 percent decrease in consumption.

This decrease in crude fiber consumption in the U.S.A. supports the hypothesis that fiber intake has decreased not so coincidentally with *increases* in colon cancer, hemorrhoids, diverticulosis, colitis, ulcerative colitis, and chronic constipation.

The best way to increase your fiber intake is to eat breads made of 100 percent whole grains, raw fruit, and to add unprocessed bran to your daily diet (it can be mixed into your regular breakfast cereal). Bran has little or no food value. We do not digest and absorb it. As it passes through the digestive tract, it accumulates liquid and swells up, providing a good amount of soft bulk that speeds bowel movements and acts to dilute levels of fat metabolites associated with carcinogen formation. Bran is also available as a food supplement in concentrated tablet form.

70. Kelp

This amazing seaweed contains more vitamins and minerals than any other food. To be more specific, kelp has vitamin B_2, niacin, choline, carotin, and algenic acid, as well as twenty-three minerals which range as follows:

Idoine	0.15–0.20%	Magnesium	0.70%
Calcium	1.20%	Sulfur	0.93%
Phosphorus	0.30%	Chlorine	12.21%
Iron	0.10%	Copper	0.0008%
Sodium	3.14%	Zinc	0.0003%
Potassium	0.63%	Manganese	0.0008%

Plus traces of: barium, boron, chromium, lithium, nickel, silver, titanium, vanadium, aluminum, strontium, and silicon.

Because of its natural iodine content, kelp has a normalizing effect on the thyroid gland. In other words, thin people with thyroid trouble can gain weight by using kelp and obese people can lose weight with it.

Homeopathic physicians use kelp for obesity, poor digestion, flatulence, and obstinate constipation; and, for the past several years, one of the most widespread fads has been the kelp, lecithin, vinegar, and B₆ diet. (See section 226.)

71. Yeast

One of the richest sources of
organic iron

It's known as nature's wonder food, and it does a lot to deserve its reputation. Yeast is an excellent source of protein and a superior source of the natural B-complex vitamins. It is one of the richest sources of organic iron and a gold mine of minerals, trace minerals, and amino acids. It has been known to help lower cholesterol (when combined with lecithin), help reverse gout, and ease the aches and pains of neuritis.

There are various sources of yeast

Brewer's yeast (from hops, a by-product of beer), sometimes called nutritional yeast.

Torula yeast grown on wood pulp used in the manufacture of paper. Or from blackstrap molasses.

Whey, a by-product of milk and cheese (best-tasting and most potent).

Liquid yeast from Switzerland and Germany, fed on herbs, honey malt, and oranges or grapefruit.

Avoid live baker's yeast! Live yeast cells deplete the B vitamins in the intestines and rob your body of all vitamins. In nutritional yeast, these live cells are heat-killed, thus preventing that depletion.

Yeast has all the major B vitamins (except B_{12}), which can be especially bred into it. It contains sixteen amino acids, fourteen or more minerals, and seventeen vitamins (except for A, E, and C). It can be considered a whole food.

Because yeast, like other protein foods, is high in phosphorus, it is advisable when taking it to add extra calcium to the diet. Phosphorus, though a coworker of calcium, can take calcium out of the body, leaving a deficiency. The remedy is simple: increase your calcium (calcium lactate assimilates well in the body). *B-complex vitamins should be taken together with yeast to be more effective. Together they work like a powerhouse.*

Yeast can be stirred into liquid, juice, or water and taken between meals. Many people who feel fatigued take a tablespoon or more in liquid and feel a return of energy within minutes, and the good effects last for several hours. Yeast can also be used as a reducing food. Stir into liquid and drink just before a meal. It takes the edge off a large appetite and saves you a lot in calories.

VI

How to Find Out What Vitamins You Really Need

72. Are You As Healthy As You Think?

TAKE THIS TEST AND SEE

Each of the following questions is designed so you can score yourself on a scale of 0 to 2 points.

$$0 = \text{NEVER} \quad 1 = \text{SOMETIMES} \quad 2 = \text{OFTEN}$$

Circle the number that applies to you, then add up your score.*

1. Do you spend a lot of time working under strong office lights?

    0 1 2

*Individuals may vary in the importance of each point scored according to genetic and other factors.

2. During the past year how often did you come down with a cold or infection?   0   1   2

3. Do you have a cocktail or two before lunch or dinner?   0   1   2

4. Do you buy many of your meals or snacks in the frozen-food section of your supermarket?   0   1   2

5. Do you smoke cigarettes?   0   1   2

6. Do you spend a lot of time in highly populated or industrialized areas?   0   1   2

7. Is lunch your first meal of the day?   0   1   2

8. Do you avoid exercising?   0   1   2

9. Do you have a sweet tooth that you can't always control?   0   1   2

10. Have you yelled or wanted to yell at your spouse or boss lately?   0   1   2

SUBTOTAL

If you are certain you are getting at least the recommended daily allowance of vitamins A, B complex, C, D, E, and minerals, subtract 1 point for each.

TOTAL

WHAT YOUR SCORE MEANS

0–6 NUTRITION WINNER:

If you're in this category, you probably feel good and generally take good care of yourself. Especially if you were able to subtract points because you're sure you're getting the vitamins A, B complex, C, D, E, and minerals you need. You know how important vitamins are to good health. And you're probably aware that though you may try to eat a balanced diet, many of today's foods have been stripped of essential nutrients through processing and cooking. To make sure you're getting the nutrients you need, you supplement your diet with vitamins.

7–14 RUNNER-UP:

If you're in this category, you may feel well, but you may not be taking as good care of yourself as you should. You may be using up more of your body's vitamin reserves than you're putting in. For instance, if you smoke, you're using up more vitamin C than people who don't smoke. If you've had a cold, your body's also used up more vitamin C which needs to be replenished. If you work under strong office lights or are a frequent television viewer, you need a larger amount of vitamin A. And as I've already mentioned, though you may try to eat a balanced diet, many foods have lost nutritional value through processing and cooking. Be sure you're putting back the nutrients your body is using up.

15–20 RISK RIDER:

Chances are if you're in this category, you may feel okay, but you're taking advantage of your body. You may be causing a vitamin deficiency without knowing it. Take a look at section 76. Because vitamin deficiencies may not become physically apparent right away, most people have no idea they're running on a deficit. If you fall into this category, I suggest you see your doctor and reexamine your diet and life-style. More than likely, you may find you need supplements.

73. Junk Foods and Nutrition

> The average person has twenty food encounters a day!

Today's families rarely breakfast together, rarely have lunch at home, and, even on weekends, eat only half of their meals as a group. In a single generation Americans have altered traditional eating habits and have become a "food-grazing" society. We now eat wherever we happen to be—and more often than not that's close to a fast-food outlet.

In twenty-five years, the per capita consumption of fast-food staples has risen dramatically. Frozen potatoes alone (used for French fries) have gone from 6.6 pounds per person to more than 36.8 pounds a year. The estimated sales for snack foods in 1978 was $3.8 billion! And since the average person has approximately twenty food encounters a day, that's a lot of easy access to junk food.

Exactly how junky, nutritionally speaking, is junk food? That depends on how much of it you eat, whether you're an adult or a child, and your own individual biologic makeup. For example, a *Consumer Reports* study of fast-food chains (including McDonalds, Burger

King, Burger Chef, Pizza Hut, Kentucky Fried Chicken, Hardee's, Arby's, and Arthur Treacher's) showed that six nutrients essential for growth and life support—biotin, folacin, pantothenic acid, total vitamin A, iron, and copper—which would usually be part of a standard diet, were in short supply in the restaurants' standard fare. For an adult with varied eating habits, this is less important than for a child for whom these meals are a way of life. Also, on the average, the fast foods tested contained more than thirty times the Recommended Daily Dietary Allowance for iodine established by the National Academy of Sciences National Research Council. And for anyone on a low-sodium diet, watch out! The specialty item at most fast-food places was almost always pre-salted.

In just about every case, fast-food meals are loaded with high carbohydrates and empty calories. And in some instances they're loaded with other things. If you've ever gotten an itchy feeling after a visit to your favorite burger haunt, it might be from the gum tragacanth (a common vegetable additive) used to bind that "special sauce" together.

All in all, though fast foods provide tasty meals at the right price, you're almost always shortchanged nutritionally.

74. What Is a Balanced Diet and Are You Eating It?

A balanced diet is something easily found in books and rarely on the table. Though nutrients

137

are widely scattered all through our food supply, soil depletion, storage, food processing, and cooking destroy many of them. Still, there are enough left to make balancing meals important. After all, supplements cannot work without food, and the better the food you eat, the more effective your supplements will be. Unfortunately, no possible "balanced" diet is likely to meet nutritional needs today.

Nevertheless, to know whether or not you are balancing your meals, you should become familiar with the four basic food groups, and the recommended number of portions that should be eaten from them each day. Serving sizes should be individually determined; smaller amounts for less active people, larger amounts for teenagers and people who do physically strenuous work.

MILK GROUP

Milk, cheese, yogurt, foods made from milk.

- 3 servings per day for a child
- 4 servings per day for a teenager
- 2 servings per day for an adult
- 4 servings per day for pregnant and lactating women

MEAT GROUP

Beef, veal, pork, lamb, fish, poultry, liver, or eggs. Dry peas, beans, soy extenders, and nuts combined with animal protein—including eggs, milk, and cheese—or grain protein can be substituted for meat serving.

- 2 servings per day
- 3 servings per day for pregnant women

FRUIT–VEGETABLE GROUP

Citrus or other fruit rich in vitamin C (or tomato juice) should be eaten daily. Dark-green, leafy, or orange vegetables and fruit should be eaten three or four times a week for vitamin A.

4 servings per day

GRAIN GROUP

Whole or enriched grains, bread in any shape, hot or cold cereals, macaroni, noodles, or other pasta.

4 servings per day

The recommended servings, as outlined by the National Research Council, are designed to supply 1,200 calories. You are expected to adjust the size of the servings to suit your own individual growth, weight, and energy needs.

75. How to Test for Deficiencies

If you're wondering whether or not you need vitamin or mineral supplementation, your best bet would be to contact a nutritionally oriented doctor. (The International Academy of Preventive Medicine, 10409 Town & Country Way, Suite 200, Houston, Texas 77024, offers a list upon request; also see section 31.) Other than that, there are a variety of "indicator" tests that should tell you enough to point you in the right supplement direction.

Dr. John M. Ellis has devised a quick early-warning test for B₆ (pyridoxine) deficiency. Extend your hand, palm up, then try to bend the two joints in your four fingers (not the knuckles of your hand) until your fingertips reach your palm. (This is not a fist, only two joints are bent.) Do this with both hands. If it is difficult, if finger joints don't allow tips to reach your palm, a pyridoxine deficiency is likely.

Betty Lee Morales, a well-known nutritionist, says that urine is a fair indicator of the B vitamins in your body. Since B vitamins are water soluble and lost each day through excretion, when your body demands more your urine will be light in color. When the urine is dark, your B demands are less. (*Note:* Many drugs, illnesses, and foods also alter urine color. This should be taken into consideration.)

Another urine test can be done at home to see if you're getting enough vitamin C:

WHAT YOU NEED

10 drops 5 percent solution of aqueous silver nitrate (can be purchased at almost any drugstore without prescription)
10 drops urine
2 paper cups
1 medicine dropper

Put ten drops of the aqueous silver nitrate solution in a paper cup. Collect a sample of your urine in the other cup, then add ten drops to the aqueous silver nitrate. Let stand two minutes. The solution will change color—from white to gray to charcoal—depending on the amount of vitamin C being excreted. The darker the solution, the more vitamin C being excreted, which means the less your body needs. You can decrease your daily intake. If the solution stays light, very little vitamin C is being excreted, which means your system is using it all and probably needs more. If this is the case, it is advisable to increase your intake.

If you want to check your mineral levels for a deficiency or an abnormally high content, have your doctor send a small amount of your hair—a tablespoon or two clipped from the back of the neck—to the Soil and Health Foundation of Emmaus, Pennsylvania, or to Parmae Laboratories, Inc., P.O. Box 35227, Dallas, Texas 75235, or to Hartley Research Labs, 1495 West Street, Provo, Utah 84601—telephone: (801) 377-5455. (Some laboratories will send results directly to individuals, others only to doctors. You can query them.)

76. Possible Warning Signs

A body in need of vitamins usually lets you know about it sooner or later. It's unlikely that any of us will come down with scurvy before realizing we need vitamin C, but more often than not our bodies are giving us clues that we just don't recognize. With the price of medical insurance rising daily, paying attention to your nutritional warning system is about the best and cheapest insurance around. Here are a few common *symptoms* that you might be ignoring—and shouldn't.

141

The supplements recommended are not intended as medical advice, only as a guide in working with your doctor.

(*Note:* NSP stands for Nutrition Starter Package. This consists of a high-potency multiple vitamin with chelated minerals, perferably time release; a vitamin C, 1,000 mg. with bioflavonoids, rutin, hesperidin, and rose hips, time release; a high-potency chelated multiple-mineral supplement. One of each to be taken with breakfast and dinner.)

POSSIBLE DEFICIENCY	ARE YOU EATING ENOUGH?	RECOMMENDED SUPPLEMENT
	Appetite Loss	
Protein	Meat, fish eggs, dairy products, soybeans, peanuts	1 B complex, 50 mg., taken with each meal. 1 B$_{12}$,
Vitamin A	Fish, liver, egg yolks, butter, cream, green leafy or yellow vegetables	2,000 mcg. (time release) with breakfast. 1 organic iron complex tablet (containing
Vitamin B$_1$	Brewer's yeast, whole grains, meat (pork or liver), nuts, legumes, potatoes	vitamin C, copper, liver, manganese, and zinc to help assimilate iron).
Vitamin C	Citrus fruits, tomatoes, potatoes, cabbage, green peppers	
Biotin	Brewer's yeast, nuts, beef liver, kidney, unpolished rice	
Phosphorus	Milk, cheese, meat, poultry, fish, cereals, nuts, legumes	
Sodium	Beef, pork, sardines, cheese, green olives, corn bread, sauerkraut	

142

Possible Deficiency	Are You Eating Enough?	Recommended Supplement
Appetite Loss		
Zinc	Vegetables, whole grains, wheat bran, wheat germ, pumpkin seeds, sunflower seeds	
Bad Breath		
Niacin	Liver, meat, fish, whole grains, legumes	1–2 tbsp. acidophilus liquid (flavored) 1 to 3 times a day. 1 chlorophyll tablet or capsule 3 times a day. 1–3 chelated zinc 50-mg. tabs 3 times a day. 1–2 multiple digestive enzyme tabs 1–3 times a day.
Body Odor		
B_{12}	Yeast, liver, beef, eggs, kidney	Same as bad breath
*Bruising Easily**		
Vitamin C	Citrus fruits, tomatoes, potatoes, cabbage, green peppers	1 C complex, 1,000 mg. (time release) with bioflavonoids, rutin, and hesperidin A.M. and P.M.
Bioflavonoids	Orange, lemon, lime, tangerine peels	

*When slight or minor injuries produce bluish, purplish discoloration of skin.

POSSIBLE DEFICIENCY	ARE YOU EATING ENOUGH?	RECOMMENDED SUPPLEMENT
	High Cholesterol	
B complex Inositol	Yeast, brewer's yeast, dried lima beans, raisins, cantaloupe	1 tbsp. acidophilus liquid 3 times daily or 3 caps 3 times daily. 2–3 tbsp. lecithin granules 3–4 times daily (used on salads or cottage cheese) or 3 1,200-mg. caps 3–4 times daily.
	Constipation	
B complex	Liver, beef, cheese, pork, kidney	1 tbsp. acidophilus liquid 3 times daily. 3–9 bran tabs daily.
	Diarrhea	
Vitamin K Niacin Vitamin F	Yogurt, alfalfa, soybean oil, fish, liver, oils, kelp Liver, lean meat, brewer's yeast, wheat germ, peanuts, dried nutritional yeast, white meat of poultry, avocado, fish, legumes, whole grain Vegetable oils, peanuts, sunflower seeds, walnuts	1 g. potassium divided over 3 meals. As a preventive 1–2 tbsp. acidophilus liquid (flavored) 3 times daily.
	Dizziness	
Manganese	Nuts, green leafy vegetables, peas, beets, egg yolks	50–100 mg. niacin 3 times a day. 400 IU vitamin E

POSSIBLE DEFICIENCY	ARE YOU EATING ENOUGH?	RECOMMENDED SUPPLEMENT
	Diarrhea	
B$_2$ (Riboflavin)	Milk, liver, kidney, yeast, cheese, fish, eggs	1–3 times a day.
	Ear Noises	
Manganese Potassium	See above. Bananas, watercress, all leafy green vegetables, citrus fruits, sunflower seeds	Same as for dizziness.
	Eye Problems*	
Vitamin A B$_2$ (Riboflavin)	See above. See above.	10,000 IU vitamin A 1–3 times daily for 5 days and stop for 2. 100 mg. B complex (time release), 1 in A.M. and P.M. 500 mg. vitamin C with bioflavonoids, rutin, and hesperidin, 1 in A.M. and P.M. 400 IU vitamin E (dry), 1 in A.M. and P.M.

*Night blindness, inability to adjust to darkness, bloodshot eyes, inflammation, burning sensations, sties.

	Fatigue*	
Zinc	Vegetables, whole-grain products, brewer's yeast, wheat bran, wheat germ, pumpkin and sunflower	1 B complex, 100 mg. (time release). 2 times daily. 1 2,000-mcg. B$_{12}$ A.M. and P.M. 1 50-mg. B$_{15}$ with

*Lassitude, weakness, no inclination for physical activity.

POSSIBLE DEFICIENCY	ARE YOU EATING ENOUGH?	RECOMMENDED SUPPLEMENT

Fatigue*

	seeds	each meal. NSP, 1 A.M. and P.M.
Carbohydrates	Cellulose	
Protein	See above.	
Vitamin A	See above.	
Vitamin B complex	See above.	
PABA	Same as B complex.	
Iron	Wheat germ, soybean flour, beef, kidney, liver, beans, clams, peaches, and molasses	
Iodine	Seafoods, dairy products, kelp	
Vitamin C	See above.	
Vitamin D	Fish liver oils, butter, egg yolk, liver, sunshine	

Gastrointestinal Problems*

Vitamin B₁ (thiamin)	See above.	25,000 IU vitamin A 1–3 times daily.
Vitamin B₂ (riboflavin)	See above.	Take for 5 days and stop for 2.
Folic acid (folacin)	Fresh green leafy vegetables, fruit, organ meats, liver, dried nutritional yeast	100 mg. B complex (time release), 1 A.M. and P.M. Multiple minerals, 1 A.M. and P.M.
PABA	Same as B complex; see above.	
Vitamin C	See above.	
Chlorine	Kelp, rye flour, ripe olives, sea greens	
Pantothenic acid	Same as B complex; see above.	

*Gastritis, gastric ulcers, gallbladder, digestive disturbances.

POSSIBLE DEFICIENCY	ARE YOU EATING ENOUGH?	RECOMMENDED SUPPLEMENT

Hair Problems

1. DANDRUFF*

POSSIBLE DEFICIENCY	ARE YOU EATING ENOUGH?	RECOMMENDED SUPPLEMENT
Vitamin B$_{12}$ (cyanocobalamin)	Liver, beef, pork, organ meats, eggs, milk and milk products	50 mcg. selenium 3 times daily. NSP, 1 A.M. and P.M.
Vitamin F	See above.	
Vitamin B$_6$	Dried nutritional yeast, liver, organ meats, legumes, whole-grain cereals, fish	
Selenium	Bran, germ of cereals, broccoli, onions, tomatoes, and tuna	

2. DULL, DRY, BRITTLE, OR GRAYING HAIR

POSSIBLE DEFICIENCY	ARE YOU EATING ENOUGH?	RECOMMENDED SUPPLEMENT
Vitamin B complex	See above.	3 vitamin-F caps with each meal. 3–6 lecithin caps with each meal NSP, 1 A.M. and P.M.
PABA	Same as B complex; see above.	
Vitamin F	See above.	
Iodine	Seafoods, iodized salt, dairy products	

*Loose flakes—dry or yellow and greasy—which fall from scalp.

3. LOSS OF HAIR

POSSIBLE DEFICIENCY	ARE YOU EATING ENOUGH?	RECOMMENDED SUPPLEMENT
Biotin	See above·	Stress B, 600 mg., 2 times daily. 1,000 mg. choline and inositol daily. 1 multiple mineral daily·
Inositol	Unrefined molasses and liver, lecithin, unprocessed whole grains, citrus fruits, brewer's yeast	
Chlorine	Sodium chloride (table salt)	
B complex with C and folic acid	See above.	

POSSIBLE DEFICIENCY	ARE YOU EATING ENOUGH?	RECOMMENDED SUPPLEMENT
Heart Palpitation		
Vitamin B$_{12}$ (cobalamin, cyancobalamin)	See above.	NSP, 1 A.M. and P.M. 100 mg. vitamin B complex (time release) A.M. and P.M. 100 mg. niacin 1–3 times daily. 3 caps lecithin 3 times daily.
High Blood Pressure		
Choline	Egg yolks, brain, heart, green leafy vegetables, yeast, liver, wheat germ	Lecithin granules, 3 tbsp. daily or 3 caps 3 times daily. NSP, 1 A.M. and P.M. Start with 100 IU vitamin E and work up to higher strengths. (See section 37.) 1–3 kelp tabs daily. 1 garlic perle 3 times daily.
Infections (high susceptibility)		
Vitamin A (carotene)	See above.	1–2 tbsp. acidophilus 3 times a day.
Pantothenic acid	Same as B complex; see above.	Vitamin A up to 100,000 IU every other day. NSP, 1 A.M. and P.M. (2–5 g. vitamin C for duration of infection.)
Insomnia		
Potassium	See above.	3 tryptophan tabs
B complex	See above.	½ hr. before bedtime. Chelated
Biotin	See above.	calcium and mag-
Calcium	Milk and milk	

148

POSSIBLE DEFICIENCY	ARE YOU EATING ENOUGH?	RECOMMENDED SUPPLEMENT
	Insomnia	
	products, meat, fish, eggs, cereal products, beans, fruit, vegetables	nesium, 1 tab 3 times daily. (See section 150.) Vitamin B_6, 50 mg. ½ hr. before bedtime. NSP, A.M. and P.M.
	Loss of Smell	
Vitamin A Zinc	See above. See above.	50 mg. chelated zinc 3 times daily (cut back to 1–2 daily when condition improves).
	Memory Loss	
B_1 (thiamine)	See above.	L-glutamine, 500 mg. 3 times daily. 50 mg. B complex A.M. and P.M. Choline, 2 g. daily in divided doses.
	Menstrual Problems	
B_{12}	See above.	NSP A.M. and P.M. 50 mg. B_6 3 times daily. 100 mg. B complex (time release) A.M. and P.M.
	Mouth Sores and Cracks	
Vitamin B_2 (riboflavin) Vitamin B_6 (pyridoxine)	See above. See above.	50 mg. B complex 3 times a day with meals. NSP A.M. and P.M.
	*Muscle Cramps**	
Vitamin B_1 (thiamin)	See above.	400 IU vitamin E (dry) 3 times

*General muscle weakness, tenderness in calf.

Possible Deficiency	Are You Eating Enough?	Recommended Supplement

Muscle Cramps*

Vitamin B$_6$ (pyridoxine)	See above.	daily. Chelated calcium and magnesium, 3 tabs 3 times daily. 100 mg. niacin 3 times daily.
Biotin	See above.	
Chlorine	See above.	
Sodium	See above.	
Vitamin D (calciferol)	See above.	

Nervousness

Vitamin B$_6$ (pyridoxine)	See above.	Stress B with C 1–3 times daily (50 mg. of all B vitamins). Approx. 660 mg. tryptophan 3 times a day and 3 tabs at bedtime. 3 chelated calcium and magnesium tabs 3 times daily. NSP A.M. and P.M.
Vitamin B$_{12}$ (cyanocobalamin)	See above.	
Niacin (nicotinic acid, niacinamide)	See above.	
PABA	See above.	
Magnesium	Green leafy vegetables, nuts, cereals, grains, seafoods	

Nosebleeds

Vitamin C	See above.	1,000 mg. vitamin C with 500 mg. rutin, hesperidin, and 500 mg. bioflavonoids (time release) A.M. and P.M.
Vitamin K	See above.	
Bioflavonoids	See above.	

Retarded Growth

Fat	Meat, butter	NSP A.M. and P.M.
Protein	See above.	
Vitamin B$_2$ (riboflavin)	See above.	
Folic acid	See above.	
Zinc	See above.	

POSSIBLE DEFICIENCY	ARE YOU EATING ENOUGH?	RECOMMENDED SUPPLEMENT
	Retarded Growth	
Cobalt	Liver, kidney, pancreas, and spleen (organ meats)	

	Skin Problems	
	1. ACNE*	
Water-solubilized vitamin A	See above.	1 multiple vitamin (without minerals) daily. 1–2 400 IU vitamin E (dry) daily, 25,000 IU vitamin A (dry), 1–2 tabs daily 6 days a week. 50 mg. chelated zinc 3 times daily with food. 1–2 tbsp· acidophilus liquid 3 times daily or 3–6 caps 3 times daily.
Vitamin B complex	See above.	

*Face blemishes, thickened skin, blackheads, whiteheads, red spots.

	2. DERMATITIS	
	(skin inflammation)	
Vitamin B$_2$ (riboflavin)	See above.	Same as above.
Vitamin B$_6$ (pyridoxine)	See above.	
Biotin	See above.	
Niacin (nicotinic acid niacinamide)	See above.	

	3. ECZEMA*	
Fat	See above.	Same as above.

*Rough, dry, scaly skin, redness and swelling, small blisters.

POSSIBLE DEFICIENCY	ARE YOU EATING ENOUGH?	RECOMMENDED SUPPLEMENT
3. ECZEMA*		
Vitamin A (carotene)	See above.	
Vitamin B complex	See above.	
Inositol	See above.	
Copper	Organ meats, oysters, nuts, dried legumes, whole-grain cereals	
Iodine	See above.	
Slow-healing Wounds and Fractures		
Vitamin C	See above.	50 mg. zinc 3 times daily. 400 IU vitamin E 3 times daily. NSP A.M. and P.M.
Softening of Bones and Teeth		
Vitamin D (calciferol)	See above.	1,000 mg. calcium, 500 mg. magnesium divided over 2 meals daily.
Calcuim	See above.	
Tremors		
Magnesium	See above.	B complex and 50 mg. B_6 3 times daily. 1,000 mg. calcium, 500 mg. magnesium divided over 3 meals daily.
Vaginal Itching		
Vitamin B_2	See above.	2 tbsp. acidophilus 3 times daily or 3–6 caps 3–4 times daily.
Water Retention		
Vitamin B_6	See above.	50 mg. B_6 3 times daily.

White Spots on Nails

Zinc	See above.	50 mg. zinc 3 times daily. Stress B with C 1–2 times daily. 1 multiple mineral 2 times daily.

77. Cravings—What They Might Mean

Cravings, which can sometimes mean allergies, are more often nature's way of letting you know that you're not getting enough of certain vitamins or minerals. Frequently these specific hungers develop because overall diet is inadequate.

Some of the most common cravings are:

Peanut Butter This is definitely among the top ten, and it's not at all surprising. Peanut butter is a rich source of B vitamins. If you find yourself dipping into the jar often, it might be because you're under stress and your ordinary B intake has become insufficient. Since 50 g. of peanut butter—a third of a cup—is 284 calories, you'll find it easier on your waistline to take a B-complex supplement if you do not want to gain weight.

Bananas When you catch yourself reaching for this fruit again and again, it could be because your body needs potassium. One medium banana has 555 mg. People taking diuretics or cortisone (which rob the body of needed potassium) often crave bananas.

Cheese If you're more a cheese luster than

153

a cheese lover, there's a good chance that your real hunger is for calcium and phosphorus. (If it's processed cheese that you've been snacking on, you've been getting aluminum, too, without knowing it.) For one thing, you might try eating more broccoli. That's high in calcium and phosphorus, and a lot lower in calories than cheese.

Apples An apple a day doesn't necessarily keep the doctor away, but it offers a lot of good things that you might be missing in other foods—calcium, magnesium, phosphorus, potassium—and is an excellent source of cholesterol-lowering pectin! If you have a tendency to eat a lot of saturated fat, it could account for your apple cravings.

Butter Most often vegetarians crave butter because of their own low-saturated-fat intake. Salted butter, on the other hand, might be craved for the salt alone.

Cola The craving for cola is most often a sugar hunger and an addiction to caffeine. (See section 197.) The beverage has no nutritive value.

Nuts If you're a little nutty about nuts, you probably could use more protein, B vitamins, or fat in your diet. If it's salted nuts you favor, you could be craving the sodium and not the nuts. You'll find that people under stress tend to eat more nuts than relaxed individuals.

Ice cream High as ice cream is in calcium, most people crave it for its sugar content. Hypoglycemics and diabetics have great hungers for it, as do people seeking to recapture the security of childhood.

Pickles If you're pregnant and want pickles,

you're probably after the salt. And if you're not pregnant and crave pickles, the reason is most likely the same. (Pickles also contain a substantial amount of potassium.)

Bacon Cravings for bacon are usually because of its fat. People on restricted diets are most susceptible to greasy binges. Unfortunately, saturated fat is not bacon's only drawback. Bacon is very high in carcinogenic nitrites. If you do indulge in bacon, be sure you're ingesting enough vitamin C and A, D, and E to counteract the nitrites.

Eggs Aside from the protein (two eggs give you 13 g.), sulfur, amino acids, and selenium protein, egg lovers might also be seeking the yolk's fat content or, paradoxically, its cholesterol-and-fat-dissolving choline.

Cantaloupe Just because you like its taste might not be the only reason you crave this melon. Cantaloupe is high in potassium and vitamin A. In fact, a quarter of a melon has 3,400 IU vitamin A. Since the melon also offers vitamin C, calcium, magnesium, phosphorus, biotin, and inositol, it's not a bad craving to give in to. There's only about 60 calories in half a melon.

Olives Whether you crave them green or black, you're likely to be after the salt. People with underactive thyroids are most often the first to reach for them.

Salt No guesswork here, it's the sodium you're after. Cravers quite possibly have a thyroid iodine deficiency or low sodium Addison's disease. Hypertensives often crave salt, and shouldn't.

Onions Cravings for spicy foods can sometimes indicate problems in the lungs or sinuses.

Chocolate Definitely one of the foremost cravings, if not *the* foremost. Chocoholics are addicted to the caffeine as well as the sugar. (There are 5 to 10 mg. of caffeine in a cup of cocoa.) If you want to kick the chocolate habit, try carob instead. (Carob, also called St. John's Bread, is made from the edible pods of the Mediterranean carob tree.)

Milk If you're still craving milk as an adult, you might need a calcium supplement. Then again, it might be the amino acids—such as tryptophan, leucine, and lysine—that your body needs. Nervous people often seek out the tryptophan in milk, since it has a very soothing effect.

Chinese food Of course it's delicious, but often it's the monosodium glutamate in the food that fosters the craving. People with salt deficiencies usually go all out for Chinese food. (MSG can cause a histamine reaction in some individuals. Headaches and flushing may occur. Most Chinese restaurants will now prepare your food without MSG if you request it.)

Mayonnaise Since this is a fatty food, it is often craved by vegetarians and people who have eliminated other fats from their diet.

Tart fruits A persistent craving for tart fruits can often indicate problems with the gallbladder or liver.

Paint and dirt Children have a tendency to eat paint and dirt. Frequently this is an indication of a calcium or vitamin-D deficiency. A hard reevaluation of your child's diet is essential, and a visit to your pediatrician is recommended.

78. Getting the Most Vitamins from Your Food

Eating the right foods doesn't necessarily mean that you're getting the vitamins they contain. Food processing, storing, and cooking can easily undermine the best nutritious intentions. To get the most from what you eat (not to mention what you spend) keep the following tips in mind.

• Wash but don't soak fresh vegetables if you hope to benefit from the B vitamins and C they contain.
• Forgo convenience and make your salads when you're ready to eat them. Fruits and vegetables cut up and left to stand lose vitamins.
• If you don't plan to eat your fresh fruit or vegetables for a few days, you're better off buying flash-frozen ones. The vitamin content of good frozen green beans will be higher than those fresh ones you've kept in your refrigerator for a week.
• Don't thaw your frozen vegetables before cooking.
• There are more vitamins in converted and parboiled rice than in polished rice, and brown rice is more nutritious than white.
• Frozen foods that you can boil in their bags offer more vitamins than the ordinary kind, and all frozen foods are preferable to canned ones.
• Cooking in copper pots can destroy vitamin C, folic acid, and vitamin E.
• Aluminum, stainless steel, glass, and enamel are the best utensils for retaining nutrients

while cooking. (Iron pots can give you the benefit of that mineral, but they will short-change you on vitamin C.)

• The shortest cooking time and the smallest amount of water are the least destructive to nutrients.

• Milk in glass containers can lose riboflavin, as well as vitamins A and D, unless kept out of the light. (Breads exposed to light can also lose these nutrients.)

• Well-browned, crusty, or toasted baked goods have less thiamine than others.

• Bake and boil potatoes in their skins to get the most vitamins from them.

• Use cooking water from vegetables to make soups, juices from meats for gravies, and syrups from canned fruits to make desserts.

• Refrain from using any baking soda when cooking vegetables if you want to benefit from their thiamine and vitamin C.

• Store vegetables and fruits in the refrigerator as soon as you bring them home from the market.

VII
Read the Label

79. The Importance of Understanding What's on Labels

All too often people buy supplements and never even look at the labels. They ask a clerk for a multivitamin and take what they are given, not realizing that they might be getting short-changed on the vitamin content. All multivitamins differ in amounts included, and the most expensive tablet is not necessarily the best. The only way to be sure you're getting the B_6, folacin, or C that you need is to read the small print on the label. Also, if you have any allergies, it's wise to check what else you're getting with your supplement. (See section 20.)

If there are words on the label that you don't understand, ask the pharmacist or vitamin clerk to explain them. If they can't, buy your supplements where someone can. And above all, remember to check the dosage you're getting. If you've been instructed to take vitamin E four times a day, it's unlikely that you want 400 IU. Vitamins and minerals come in different strengths. Be sure you're getting what you ask for—and need. Not understanding labels can often negate a lot of vitamin benefits.

80. How Does That Measure Up?

> IU, RE, MG, MCG—a little
> can mean a lot.

The terminology for measuring vitamin activity is not as confusing as you might think. Fat-soluble vitamins (A, E, D, and K) are usually measured in International Units (IU). Recently, though, an expert committee of the Food and Agriculture Organization/World Health Organization (FAO/WHO) decided to change this order of measurement for vitamin A. Instead of using International Units, they proposed that vitamin A be evaluated in terms of retinol equivalents (RE), that is, the equivalent weight of retinol (vitamin A_1, alcohol) *actually absorbed and converted.*

Retinol equivalents come out to about five times less than International Units (IU). Recommended allowances of 5,000 IU for a male between the ages of twenty-three and fifty would only be 1,000 RE; 4,000 IU for similarly aged females would only be 800 RE.

Most other vitamins and minerals are measured in milligrams (mg.) and micrograms (mcg.). If you know that 1 g. equals .035 ounce, that it takes 28.35 g. to equal 1 ounce (and 1 fluid ounce equals 2 tablespoons), you'll have a better idea of just how much—or rather, how little—it takes for vitamins and minerals to do their job. The following table is a handy guide to refer to:

WHAT'S WHAT IN WEIGHTS AND MEASURES

Metric Measure

1 kilogram equals 1,000 grams
1 gram equals 1,000 milligrams
1 milligram equals 1/1,000th part of a gram
1 microgram equals 1/1,000th part of a milligram
1 gamma equals 1 microgram

Avoirdupois Weight

16 ounces equal 1 pound
7,000 grains equal 1 pound
453.6 grams equal 1 pound
1 ounce av. equals 437.5 grains
1 ounce av. equals 28.35 grams

Conversion Factors

1 gram equals 15.4 grains
1 grain equals 0.065 grams (65 milligrams)
1 ounce apothecary equals 31.1 grams
1 fluid ounce equals 29.8 cc.
1 fluid ounce equals 480 minims

Liquid Measure

1 drop equals 1 minim
1 minim equals 0.06 cc.
15 minims equal 1.0 cc.
4 cc. equals 1 fluid dram
30 cc. equals 1 fluid ounce

Household Measure

1 teaspoon equals 4 cc. equals 1 fluid dram
1 tablespoon equals 15 cc. equals ½ fluid ounce
½ pint equals 240 cc. equals 8 fluid ounces

Abbreviations

AMDR	Adult Minimum Daily Requirement
USP Unit	United States Pharmacopia
IU	International Unit
MDR	Minimum Daily Requirement
mg.	milligram
mcg.	microgram
g.	gram
gr.	grain

81. Breaking the RDA Code

Many people are bewildered by the variances between vitamin standards listed as RDA, U.S. RDA, and MDR. It becomes much less confusing when you understand that they are not the same thing.

RDA (*Recommended Daily Dietary Allowances*) came into being in 1941, when the Food and Nutrition Board of the National Research Council of the Academy of Sciences was established by the government to safeguard public health. The RDA are not formulated to cover the needs of those who are ill—they are not therapeutic and are meant strictly for healthy individuals—nor do they take into account nutrient losses that occur during processing and preparation. They are *estimates* of nutritional needs necessary to ensure satisfactory growth of children and the prevention of nutrient depletion in adults. *They are not meant to be optimal intakes, nor are they recommendations for an ideal diet.* They are not average requirements but recommendations intended to meet the needs of those *healthy* people with the highest requirements.

U.S. RDA (*U.S. Recommended Daily Allowances*) were formulated by the Food and Drug Administration (FDA) to be used as the *legal* standards for food labeling in regard to nutrient content. (The RDA were used as the basis for the U.S. RDA.) Calories and ten nutrients must be listed on food labels—protein, carbohydrate, fat, vitamin A, vitamin C, thiamin, riboflavin, niacin, calcium, and iron. Because the U.S. RDA are based on the highest values of the RDA, the former is frequently higher than the basic needs of most healthy people, though very few individuals today fall into that hypothetical category. Individuals vary by wide margins, and stress and illness, past and present, affect everyone differently. As far as I am concerned (and many other leading nutritionists), the RDA and U.S. RDA are woefully inadequate.

MDR (*Minimum Daily Requirements*) were the first set of standards established by the

FDA and have been revised and replaced by the U.S. RDA.

U.S. RECOMMENDED DAILY ALLOWANCES (U.S. RDA)

	Adults and Children (four years and over)
Protein*	
Protein quality equal to or greater than casein	45 g.
Protein quality less than casein	65 g.
Vitamin A*	5,000 IU
Vitamin C (ascorbic acid)*	60 mg.
Thiamine (vitamin B_1)*	1.5 mg.
Riboflavin (vitamin B_2)*	1.7 mg.
Niacin*	20 mg.
Calcium*	1.0 g.
Iron*	18 mg.
Vitamin D	400 IU
Vitamin E	30 IU
Vitamin B_6	2.0 mg.
Folic acid (folacin)	0.4 mg.
Vitamin B_{12}	6 mcg.
Phosphorus	1.0 g.
Iodine	150 mcg.
Magnesium	400 mg.
Zinc	15 mg.
Copper	2 mg.
Biotin	0.3 mg.
Pantothenic acid	10 mg.

*These nutrients *must* appear on nutrition labels. The other nutrients *may* appear.

82. What to Look For

As noted, when buying minerals, look for *chelated* on the label. Only 10 percent of ordinary minerals will be assimilated by the body, but when combined with amino acids in chelation, the assimilation is three to five times more efficient.

Hydrolyzed means water dispersible. *Hydrolyzed protein-chelate* means the supplement is in its most easily assimilated form.

Predigested protein is protein that has already been broken down and can go straight to the bloodstream.

Cold pressed is important to look for when buying oil or oil capsules. It means vitamins haven't been destroyed by heat, and that the oil, extracted by cold-pressed methods, remains polyunsaturated.

VIII

Balancing Your Vitamin Act

83. Balancing Vitamins and Minerals Is Essential

Vitamins and minerals do not work alone. We need minerals if we want our vitamins to be effective, just as we need balance if we want our minerals to be effective. Too much of even good things can be bad. For example:

Too much phosphorus can cost you calcium.
Too much sodium and you can lose potassium.
Too much zinc and you can suffer iron and copper loss.
Too much copper and you can deplete your zinc.

Too much vitamin D can raise calcium levels too high.

Too much vitamin C can cost you B_{12} and folic acid.

Too much choline can cause B_6 deficiency.

84. The B-Vitamin Balance

There are twenty-two known vitamins in the B-complex group, and they are synergistic; they work better together than individually. Just as an undersupply of one can sometimes cause another to fill in, an oversupply of any one can cause deficiencies in the others.

It is best to obtain all the B vitamins together, either in the foods you eat or by combining them with a balanced B-complex supplement. B_1, B_2, and B_6 should be taken in equal strengths, as should choline and inositol. It's remarkable how foolish we can be in regard to nutrition, removing all the B vitamins from our flour and whole-grain cereals and then returning only a few of them, which could cause imbalances that might lead to unnecessary deficiencies.

85. What You Shouldn't Take With . . .

Vitamin A should *not* be taken with mineral oil.

Vitamin C should *not* be taken with ginseng.

Vitamin E should *not* be taken with inorganic iron (ferrous sulfate) or chlorine.

167

86. How to Get the Most from Your Supplements

Supplements taken together are often more potent than any one of them taken separately. Here are some of the best combinations:

Vitamin A works best with ... B complex, vitamin D, vitamin E, calcium, phosphorus, and zinc.

Vitamin D works best with ... vitamin A, vitamin C, choline, calcium, and phosphorus.

Vitamin E works best with ... B complex, inositol, vitamin C, and manganese.

Vitamin C (ascorbic acid) works best with ... bioflavonoids, calcium, and magnesium.

Folic acid (folacin) works best with ... B complex and vitamin C.

Niacin works best with ... vitamin B_1, vitamin B_2, and vitamin C.

Vitamin B_1 (thiamine) works best with ... B complex, B_2, folic acid, niacin, vitamin C, and vitamin E.

Vitamin B_2 (riboflavin) works best with ... vitamin B_6, vitamin C, and niacin.

Vitamin B_6 (pyridoxine) works best with ... vitamin B_1, vitamin B_2, pantothenic acid, vitamin C, and magnesium.

Vitamin B_{12} (cyanocobalamin) works best with ... vitamin B_6, vitamin C, folic acid, choline, inositol, and potassium.

Calcium works best with ... vitamin A, vitamin C, vitamin D, iron, magnesium, and phosphorus.

Phosphorus works best with ... calcium, vitamin A, vitamin D, iron, and manganese.

Iron works best with ... vitamin B_{12}, folic acid, vitamin C, and calcium.

Magnesium works best with ... vitamin B_6, vitamin C, vitamin D, calcium, and phosphorus.

Zinc works best with ... vitamin A, calcium, and phosphorus.

IX

Protein—and the Great Macronutrient Misunderstanding

87. How Much Protein Do You Need, Really?

Everyone's protein requirements differ, depending on a variety of factors including health, age, and size. Actually, the larger and younger you are, the more you need. To estimate your own personal daily recommended allowance, see the chart below.

AGE	1–3	4–6	7–10	11–14	15–18	19 and over
POUND KEY	0.82	0.68	0.55	0.45	0.40	0.36

- Find the pound key under your age group.
- Multiply that number by your weight.
- The result will be your daily protein requirement in grams.

Example: You weigh 100 pounds and are thirty-
three years old.
Your pound key is 0.36.
0.36 × 100 = 36 g.—your daily protein requirement.

An average minimum protein requirement is
around 45 g. a day. That's 15 g. or about half
an ounce per meal. Make sure you get enough
at breakfast.

88. Types of Protein—What's the Difference?

All proteins are not the same, though they're
manufactured from the same twenty amino
acids. They have different functions and work
in different areas of the body.

There are basically two types of protein—
complete protein and incomplete protein.

Complete protein provides the proper balance
of eight necessary amino acids that build tissues, and is found in foods of animal origin such
as meats, poultry, seafood, eggs, milk, and
cheese.

Incomplete protein lacks certain essential
amino acids and is not used efficiently when
eaten alone. However, when it is combined with
small amounts of animal-source protein, it becomes complete. It is found in seeds, nuts, peas,
grains, and beans.

Mixing complete and incomplete proteins can
give you better nutrition than either one alone.
A good rice and beans dish with some cheese

171

can be just as nourishing, less expensive, and lower in fat than a steak.

89. Protein Myths

A lot of people seem to think that protein is nonfattening. This misconception has frustrated many a determined dieter who forgoes bread but eats healthy portions of steak and wonders where the weight is coming from. The fact is

- 1 g. protein = 4 calories
- 1 g. carbohydrate = 4 calories
- 1 g. fat = 9 calories

In other words, protein and carbohydrate have the same gram-for-gram calorie count.

It is also thought that protein can burn up fat. This is another erroneous assumption that leaves dieters staring incomprehensibly at their scales. It just is not true that the more protein you eat the thinner you'll get. And, believe it or not, one homemade beef taco or a slice of cheese pizza will give you more protein than two eggs or four slices of bacon or even a whole cup of milk. (Of course, if the taco or pizza are made with all sorts of additives, you're better off taking a cut in protein and sticking with the eggs.)

90. Protein Supplements

> Two tablespoons of supplement
> equal the protein in a three-ounce steak.

For anyone who isn't able to get his or her daily protein requirement from whole food, protein supplements are helpful. The best formulas are derived from soybeans, which contain all the essential amino acids. They come in liquid and powdered form, are available without carbohydrates or fats, and generally supply about 26 g. of protein an ounce (two tablespoons). That would be about the same amount of protein you get from a three-ounce T-bone.

Supplements can easily be added to beverages and foods. Texturized vegetable protein can be added to ground beef to extend and enhance hamburgers, which will be more economical and better for you because of the cut in saturated fat.

X

Fat and Fat Manipulators

91. Lipotropics—What Are They?

Methionine, choline, inositol, and betaine are all lipotropics, which means their prime function is to prevent abnormal or excessive accumulation of fat in the liver.

Lipotropics also increase the liver's production of lecithin, which keeps cholesterol more soluble, detoxifies the liver, and increases resistance to disease by helping the thymus gland carry out its functions.

92. Who Needs Them and Why

We all need lipotropics, some of us more than others. Anyone on a high-protein diet falls into the latter category. Methionine and choline are *necessary* to detoxify the amines that are by-products of protein metabolism.

Because nearly all of us consume too much fat (the average consumption in the United States is now 40 to 45 percent of total calories), and a good part of that is saturated fat, lipotropics are indispensable. By helping the liver produce lecithin, they're helping to keep cholesterol from forming dangerous deposits in blood vessels, lessening chances of heart attacks, arteriosclerosis, and gallstone formation as well.

> Lipotropics keep cholesterol
> moving safely.

We also need lipotropics to stay healthy, since they aid the thymus in stimulating the production of antibodies, the growth and action of phagocytes (which surround and gobble up invading viruses and microbes), and in destroying foreign or abnormal tissue.

93. The Cholesterol Story

Like everything else, there's a good and bad side to fats. The general misconception that all of them are bad for you, prevalent as it may be, simply is not true. And the most maligned of all is cholesterol.

Practically everyone knows that cholesterol can be responsible for arteriosclerosis, heart attacks, a variety of illnesses, but very few are aware of the ways that it is *essential* to health.

At least two-thirds of your body cholesterol is produced by the liver or in the intestine. It is found there as well as in the brain, the adrenals, and nerve fiber sheaths. And when it's good, it's very, very good:

• Cholesterol in the skin is converted to essential vitamin D when touched by the sun's ultraviolet rays.
• Cholesterol aids in the metabolism of carbohydrates. (The more carbohydrates ingested, the more cholesterol produced.)
• Cholesterol is a prime supplier of life-essential adrenal steroid hormones, such as cortisone, and sex hormones.

New research shows that cholesterol behaves differently depending on the protein to which it is bound. Lipoproteins are the factors in our blood which transport cholesterol. Low-density lipoproteins (LDL) carry about 65 percent of blood cholesterol, very-low-density lipoproteins (VLDL) about 15 percent, and do seem to bear a correlation to heart disease. But high-density lipoproteins (HDL), which carry about 20 percent, appear to have the opposite effect. HDL are composed principally of lecithin, whose detergent action breaks up cholesterol and can transport it easily through the blood without clogging arteries. Essentially, the higher your HDL, the lower your chances of developing symptoms of heart disease.

It's interesting to note that females, who live eight years longer than males on the average, have higher HDL levels, and, surprisingly, so do moderate alcohol drinkers.

> Eggs might not be as bad
> as you thought.

It is also worth mentioning that though the egg consumption in the United States is one-half of what it was in 1945, there has *not* been a comparable decline in heart disease. And though the American Heart Association deems eggs hazardous, a diet without them can be equally hazardous. Not only do eggs have the most perfect protein components of any food, but they contain lecithin, which aids in fat assimilation. And, most important, they *raise* HDL levels!

94. How to Raise and Lower Cholesterol Levels

RAISE CHOLESTEROL	LOWER CHOLESTEROL
Cigarettes	Eggplant
Food additives such as BHT	Onions (raw or cooked)
Pollutants such as PCBs	Garlic
Coffee	Yogurt (even made from whole milk)
Stress	
The pill	Pectin (unpeeled apple, scraped apple, white membrane of citrus fruits)
Refined sugar	
	Soybeans

For cholesterol watchers, a meal of light-meat turkey is a good choice, especially since no more than 300 mg. of cholesterol a day are recommended for the average person. Three ounces of light-meat turkey have only about

177

67 mg. cholesterol (though the same amount of dark meat has 75 mg.). Be careful of turkey liver, though; one cup of it, chopped, has about 839 mg. And remember, vegetables are cholesterol-free without butter.

XI

Carbohydrates and Enzymes

95. Why Carbohydrates Are Necessary

Carbohydrates, the scourge of misinformed dieters, are the main suppliers of our body's energy. During digestion, starches and sugars, the principal kinds of carbohydrates, are broken down into glucose, better known as blood sugar. This blood sugar provides the essential energy for our brain and central nervous system.

You need carbohydrates in your daily diet so that vital tissue-building protein is not wasted for energy when it might be needed for repair.

> They have the same calories as protein.

If you eat too many carbohydrates, more than can be converted into glucose or glycogen (which is stored in liver and muscles), the result, as we know all too well, is fat. When the body needs more fuel, the fat is converted back to glucose and you lose weight.

Don't be too down on carbohydrates. They're as important for good health as other nutrients —and gram for gram they have the same 4 calories as protein. Though no official requirement exists, a minimum of 50 g. daily is recommended to avoid ketosis, an acid condition of the blood that can happen when your own fat is used primarily for energy.

96. The Truth About Enzymes

Enzymes are necessary for the digestion of food, releasing valuable vitamins, minerals, and amino acids which keep us alive and healthy.

Enzymes are catalysts, meaning they have the power to cause an internal action without themselves being changed or destroyed in the process.

Enzymes are destroyed under certain heat conditions.

Enzymes are best obtained from uncooked or unprocessed fruits, vegetables, eggs, meats, and fish.

Each enzyme acts upon a specific food; one cannot substitute for the other. A deficiency, shortage, or even the absence of one single enzyme can mean the difference between sickness and health.

Enzymes that end in *-ase* are named by the

food substance they act upon. For example, with phosphorus the enzyme is called phosphatase; with sugar (sucrose) it is known as sucrase.

Pepsin is a vital digestive enzyme that breaks up the proteins of ingested food, splitting them into usable amino acids. Without pepsin, protein could not be used to build healthy skin, strong skeletal structure, rich blood supply, and strong muscles.

Renin is a digestive enzyme which causes coagulation of milk, changing its protein, casein, into a usable form in the body. Renin releases the valuable minerals from milk, calcium, phosphorus, potassium, and iron that are used by the body to stabilize the water balance, strengthen the nervous system, and produce strong teeth and bones.

Lipase splits fat, which is then utilized to nourish the skin cells, protect the body against bruises and blows, and ward off the entrance of infectious virus cells and allergic conditions.

Hydrochloric acid in the stomach works on tough foods such as fibrous meats, vegetables, and poultry. It digests protein, calcium, and iron. Without HCl, problems such as pernicious anemia, gastric carcinoma, congenital achlorhydria, and allergies can develop. Because stress, tension, anger, and anxiety before eating, as well as deficiencies of some vitamins (B complex primarily) and minerals, can all cause a lack of HCl, more of us are short of it than realize it. If you think that you have an over-acid problem or heartburn, for which you are dosing yourself with an antacid such as Maalox,

Di-Gel, Tums, Rolaids, or Alka-Seltzer, you are probably unaware that *the symptoms of having too little acid are exactly the same as having too much,* in which case the taking of antiacids, could be the worst possible thing for you to do.

Dr. Alan Nittler, author of *A New Breed of Doctor,* has stated emphatically that everyone over the age of forty should be using a HCl supplement.

Betaine HCl and glutamic acid HCl are the best forms of commercially available hydrochloric acid.

97. The Twelve Tissue Salts and Their Functions

Tissue salts are inorganic mineral components of your body's tissues. They are also known as Schuessler biochemical cell salts, after Dr. W.H. Schuessler, who isolated them in the late nineteenth century. Dr. Schuessler found that if the body was deficient in any of these salts, illness occurred, and that if the deficiency was corrected, the body could heal itself. In other words, tissue salts are *not a cure,* but merely a remedy.

The twelve tissue salts are:

Fuoride of lime (calc. fluor.)—Part of all the connective tissues in your body. An imbalance can be the cause of varicose veins, late dentition, muscle tendon strain, carbuncles, and cracked skin.

Phosphate of lime (calc. phos.)—Found in

all your body's cells and fluids, an important element in gastric juices as well as bones and teeth. An imbalance or deficiency can be the cause of cold hands and feet, numbness, hydrocele, sore breasts, and night sweats.

Sulfate of lime (calc. sulf.)—A constituent of all connective tissue in minute particles, as well as in the cells of the liver. An imbalance or deficiency can be the cause of skin eruptions, deep abscesses, or chronic oozing ulcers.

Phosphate of iron (ferr. phos.)—Part of your blood and other body cells, with the exception of nerves. An imbalance or deficiency can be the cause of continuous diarrhea or, paradoxically, constipation. It has also been used as a remedy for nosebleeds and excessive menses.

Chloride of potash (kali. mur.)—Found in lining and under the surface body cells. An imbalance or deficiency can be the cause of granulation of the eyelids, blistering eczema, and warts.

Sulfate of potash (kali. sulf.)—The cells that form your skin and internal organ linings interact with this salt. An imbalance or deficiency can be the cause of skin eruptions, a yellow coating on the back of the tongue, feelings of heaviness, and pains in the limbs.

Potassium phosphate (kali. phos.)—Found in all your body tissues, particularly nerve, brain, and blood cells. An imbalance or deficiency can be the cause of improper fat digestion, poor memory, anxiety, insomnia, and a faint, rapid pulse.

Phosphate of magnesia (mag. phos.)—Another mineral element of bones, teeth, brain, nerves, blood, and muscle cells. An imbalance

183

or deficiency can be the cause of cramps, neuralgia, shooting pains, and colic.

Chloride of soda (nat. mur.)—Regulates the amount of moisture in the body and carries moisture to cells. An imbalance or deficiency can be the cause of salt cravings, hay fever, watery discharges from eyes and nose.

Phosphate of soda (nat. phos.)—Emulsifies fatty acids and keeps uric acid soluble in the blood. An imbalance or deficiency can be the cause of jaundice, sour breath, an acid or coppery taste in the mouth.

Sulfate of soda (nat. sulf.)—A slight irritant to tissues and functions as a stimulant for natural secretions. An imbalance or deficiency can be the cause of low fevers, edema, depression, and gallbladder disorders.

Silicic acid (silicea)—Part of all connective tissue cells, as well as those of the hair, nails, and skin. A deficiency or imbalance can be the cause of poor memory, carbuncles, falling hair, and ribbed, ingrowing nails. Eating whole-grain products should supply the normal need for this tissue salt.

XII

Vitamin "Yeses" and "Nos" You Should Know

98. Cautions

Though we all know that vitamins are good for us, there are times, situations, and metabolic conditions where caution and special adjustments are advised. I recommend you look over the following list carefully for your own well-being and in order to get the most from your vitamins.

• Chronic hypervitaminosis A can occur in patients receiving megadoses as treatment for dermatological conditions.
• A deficiency of vitamin A can lead to loss of vitamin C.
• An oversupply of vitamin B_1 (thiamine) can

affect thyroid and insulin production and might cause B$_6$ deficiency, as well as loss of other B vitamins.

• Prolonged ingestion of any B vitamin can result in significant depletion of the others.

• Pregnant women should check with their doctors before taking sustained doses of over 50 mg. of vitamin B$_6$ (pyridoxine).

• B$_6$ should not be taken by anyone under L-dopa treatment for Parkinson's disease.

• Because vitamin D promotes absorption of calcium, a large excess of stored vitamin D can cause too much calcium in the blood (hypercalcemia).

• Don't eat raw egg whites. They deactivate the body's biotin.

• It is possible that large amounts of vitamin C might reverse the anticoagulant activity of the blood thinner warfarin, commonly prescribed as the drug Coumadin.

• Diabetics and heart patients should check with their doctors, because vitamin C might necessitate a lower dosage of pills.

• Megadoses of vitamin C wash out B$_{12}$ and folic acid, so be sure you are taking at least the daily requirement of both.

• Excessive doses of choline, taken over a long period of time, may produce a deficiency of vitamin B$_6$.

• If you have a heart disorder, check with your physician for the proper vitamin-D dosage to take.

• Vitamin E should be used cautiously by anyone with an overactive thyroid, diabetes, high blood pressure, or rheumatic heart disease. (If you have any of these conditions, start at a very low dosage and build up gradually by 100 IU daily each month to between 400 and 800 IU.)

• Rheumatic heart fever sufferers should know that they have an imbalance between the two sides of their hearts and large vitamin-E doses can increase the imbalance and worsen the condition. (Before using supplements, consult your physician.)

• Vitamin E can elevate blood pressure in hypertensives, but if supplementation is started with a low dosage and increased slowly, the end result will be an eventual lowering of the pressure through the vitamin's diuretic properties.

• Diabetics have been able to reduce their insulin levels with E. Check with your physician.

• Decreases in vitamin E should be gradual, too.

• An excessive intake of folic acid can mask symptoms of pernicious anemia.

• High doses of folic acid for extended periods of time are not recommended for anyone with a medical history of convulsive disorders or hormone-related cancer.

• Folic acid and PABA might inhibit the effectiveness of sulfonamides, such as Gantrisin.

• Megadoses of vitamin K can build up and cause a red cell breakdown and anemia.

• Patients on the blood thinner Dicumarol should be aware that synthetic K could counteract the effectiveness of the drug. Conversely, the drug inhibits the absorption of natural vitamin K.

- Sweats and flushes can occur from too much vitamin K.
- Niacin should be used cautiously by anyone with severe diabetes, glaucoma, peptic ulcers, or with impaired liver function.
- Do not give niacin to your dog or cat; it causes flushing and sweating and greatly discomforts the animal. Do not supplement a pet's diet with vitamins A or D unless your vet specifically advises it.
- Excessive amounts of PABA (Para-aminobenzoic acid) in certain individuals can have a negative effect on the liver, kidneys, and heart.
- Iron should not be taken by anyone with sickle-cell anemia, hemochromatosis, or thalassemia.
- If your iron supplement is ferrous sulfate, you're losing vitamin E.
- Large quantities of caffeine can inhibit iron absorption.
- Anyone with kidney malfunction should not take more than 300 mg. of magnesium on a daily basis.
- Too much manganese will reduce utilization of the body's iron.
- High doses of manganese can cause motor difficulties and weakness in certain individuals.
- Diets high in fat increase phosphorus absorption and lower your calcium levels.
- If you take cortisone and aldosterone drugs, such as Aldactone and prednisone, you lose potassium and retain sodium. Check with your physician for proper supplements.
- Excessive perspiration can cause a depletion of sodium.

- Too much sodium can cause a potassium loss.
- Excessive zinc intakes can result in iron and copper losses.
- If you add zinc to your diet, be sure you're getting enough vitamin A.
- Anyone suffering from Wilson's disease is susceptible to copper toxicity.
- Too much cobalt may cause an unwanted enlargement of the thyroid gland.
- Anyone taking thyroid medication should be aware that kelp also affects that gland. If you have been using both, a consultation with your doctor and retesting are advised. You might need *less* prescription medicine than you think.
- Large amounts of raw cabbage can cause an iodine deficiency and throw off thyroid production in individuals with existing low-iodine intakes.
- Milk that contains synthetic vitamin D can deplete the body of magnesium.
- Heavy coffee and tea drinkers—cola drinkers, too—should be aware that large caffeine ingestion creates an inositol shortage.
- Inform your doctor if you're taking large amounts of vitamin C. C can change results of lab tests for sugar in the blood and urine and give false negative results in tests for blood in stool specimens.
- Don't engage in strenuous physical activity within four hours after taking vitamin A if you want optimum absorption.
- Copper has a tendency to accumulate in the blood and deplete the brain's zinc supplies.
- Tryptophan should not be taken with protein; use juice or water to swallow tablets, not milk.

189

99. Questions and Answers About Vitamin Safety

Does a strong odor mean spoilage, and if so can be vitamins be harmful? Strong odors don't necesstrily signify spoilage, but it is possible. (If you have been keeping your vitamins in sunlight and warmth it is more than possible, it's probable.) But even if your vitamins have spoiled, they won't harm you. The worst that can happen is that they lose their effectiveness.

There is sometimes an alcohol smell in certain vitamin preparations. Are they still safe for consumption? Alcohol is used as a drying agent to prevent any moisture contamination. Occasionally, when the product is packed too quickly, some of the alcohol smell remains. Your vitamins are perfectly safe. Put a few kernels of rice in the bottle. They will absorb the moisture and the smell.

Are cracked vitamins safe to take? Poor tablet coating causes the cracks, but the vitamins are still effective and safe.

I take a multiple vitamin and mineral tablet as well as a multiple mineral pill twice a day. Can I safely take a zine supplement, or am I overdoing my minerals? Check your labels and see how much you're already getting. 50 mg. of zinc is usually sufficient. You don't need any extra. Though zinc is virtually nontoxic, there have been ill effects from intakes over 150 mg.

Is it true that large amounts of vitamin C can cause urological problems? Nobel Prize Winner Linus Pauling says that vitamin C is harmless and takes 13,000 mg. daily. I take 4,000 mg. daily myself, and have only good to report. There might be a few individuals whose systems respond negatively to large amounts of vitamin C, but they're definitely a minority. My feeling is that the benefits of vitamin C far outweigh the concerns. If you have urological problems, check with your doctor, or an ortho-molecular physician.

How can I be sure there is no hidden sugar in my vitamin supplements? You can't, unless you only purchase vitamins where the label plainly states that they contain no sugar or starch. Beware of shiny coatings. These are usually sugar coated. Remember, the label is not required to say what the vitamin coating consists of. Your best bet is to buy from a store that handles quality vitamins stating *all* their ingredients.

If I take a multiple vitamin and additional folic acid, am I in danger? The FDA has limited folic acid without a prescription to strengths under 1,000 mcg. A common daily dose is 408 to 800 mcg., and chances are you're not even getting that. Even if you are getting more, there's no reason to worry. Folic acid is a B vitamin, and like all B vitamins it is water soluble and not stored in the body.

I see that there is vitamin D in my mineral formula. If I take a multivitamin as well, isn't

191

it unsafe? No. The FDA dropped its suit for restriction of vitamin D because they could not prove that it was harmful in logical strength. Vitamin D is very necessary to assimilate calcium. Also, if we live in urban areas, polluted by smog, our bodies are not manufacturing enough vitamin D.

I've heard that dolomite is good for healing broken bones. I'm taking multivitamin capsules twice a day already, but can I also take dolomite? Dolomite is an excellent source of calcium and magnesium, and your multivitamin —even with minerals—is not only safe but recommended. Just make sure you're getting the proper calcium-magnesium balance (twice as much calcium as magnesium).

Are the dyes used in vitamin coatings natural or artificial, and how can I tell? Unfortunately, a lot of synthetic vitamins use coal-tar dyes in their coatings—and keep it a secret. These dyes are not necessarily harmful, but they can cause allergic reactions. My advice is to play it safe and buy natural vitamins that have no artificial adulterants—and say so!

What vitamins can I overdose on? There are only two vitamins where toxicity should be a concern—*synthetic vitamin A* and *synthetic vitamin D*. Fortunately, the FDA has limited the potency of these vitamins for over-the-counter sale. My own recommendation regarding these vitamins is common sense. If you are taking large doses of A and D, take them for five days and stop for two, or take them every other day so that they don't build up in your system.

What can happen if I take lecithin and don't really need it? Lecithin is a natural food. Forty percent of the brain is lecithin. The average American eats a hundred pounds of saturated fats per person per year, so we need poly-unsaturates—which is what lecithin is. And since the principal composition of high-density lipoprotein (HDL) is lecithin—and HDL is capable of making cholesterol soluble by its detergent action—its presence in your diet is purely beneficial, substantially *lowering* the risk of arteriosclerosis.

XIII

Translating from Vitamin-ese

100. Glossary

absorption: the process by which nutrients are passed into the bloodstream

acetate: a derivative of acetic acid

acetic acid: used as a synthetic flavoring agent, one of the first food additives (vinegar is approximately 4 to 6 percent acetic acid); it is found naturally in cheese, coffee, grapes, peaches, raspberries, and strawberries. Generally Recognized As Safe (GRAS) when used only in packaging

acetone: a colorless solvent for fat, oils, and waxes that is obtained by fermentation (inhalation can irritate lungs, and large amounts have a narcotic effect)

acid: a water-soluble substance with sour taste

194

adrenals: the glands, located above each kidney, that manufacture adrenaline

alkali: an acid-neutralizing substance (sodium bicarbonate is an alkali used for excess acidity in foods)

Alzheimer's disease: a progressively degenerative disease, involved with loss of memory, that new research indicates might be helped with extra choline

amino acids: the organic compounds from which proteins are constructed; there are twenty-two known amino acids, but only nine are indispensable nutrients for man—histidine, isoleucine, leucine, lysine, total S-containing amino acids, total aromatic amino acids, threonine, tryptophan, and valine

amino acid chelates: chelated minerals that have been produced by many of the same processes nature uses to chelate minerals in the body; in the digestive tract, nature surrounds the elemental minerals with amino acid, permitting them to be absorbed into the bloodstream

antioxidant: a substance that can protect another substance from oxidation; added to foods to keep oxygen from changing the food's color

antitoxin: an antibody formed in response to, and capable of neutralizing, a poison of biologic origin

assimilation: the process whereby nutrients are used by the body and changed into living tissue

ATP: a molecule called adenosine triphosphate, the fuel of life, a nucleotide—building block of nucleic acid—that produces biological energy with B₁, B₂, B₃, and pantothenic acid

avidin: a protein in egg white capable of inactivating biotin

bariatrician: a weight-control doctor

BHA: butylated hydroxyanisole; a preservative and antioxidant used in many products; insoluble in water; can be toxic to the kidneys

BHT: butylated hydroxytoluene; a solid, white crystalline antioxidant used to retard spoilage of many foods; can be more toxic to the kidney than its nearly identical chemical cousin, BHA

bioflavonoids: usually from orange and lemon rinds, these citrus-flavored compounds needed to maintain healthy blood-vessel walls are widely available in plants, citrus fruits, and rose hips; known as vitamin P complex

calciferol: a colorless, odorless crystalline material, insoluble in water; soluble in fats; a synthetic form of vitamin D made by irradiating ergosterol with ultraviolet light ·

calcium gluconate: an organic form of calcium

capillary: a minute blood vessel, one of many that connect the arteries and veins

carcinogen: a cancer-causing substance

carotene: an orange-yellow pigment occurring in many plants, and capable of being converted into vitamin A in the body

casein: the protein in milk that has become the standard by which protein quality is measured

catabolism: the metabolic change of nutrients

or complex substances into simpler compounds, accompanied by a release of energy

catalyst: a substance that modifies, especially increases, the rate of chemical reaction without being consumed or changed in the process

chelation: a process by which mineral substances are changed into easily digestible form

chronic: of long duration; continuing; constant

coenzyme: the major portion, though nonprotein, part of an enzyme; usually a B vitamin

collagen: the primary organic constituent of bone, cartilage, and connective tissue (becomes gelatin through boiling)

congenital: condition existing at birth, not hereditary

dehydration: a condition resulting from an excessive loss of water from the body

desiccated: dried; preserved by removing moisture

diuretic: tending to increase the flow of urine from the body

DNA: deoxyribonucleic acid; the nucleic acid in chromosomes that is part of the chemical basis for hereditary characteristics

enteric coated: a tablet coated so that it dissolves in the intestine, not in the stomach (which is acid)

enzyme: a protein substance found in living cells that brings about chemical changes; necessary for digestion of food

excipient: any inert substance used as a dilutent or vehicle for a drug

FDA: Food and Drug Administration

fibrin: an insoluble protein that forms the necessary fibrous network in the coagulation of blood

free-radicals: highly reactive chemical fragments that can produce an irritation of artery walls, start the arteriosclerotic process if vitamin E is not present; generally harmful

fructose: a natural sugar occurring in fruits and honey; called fruit sugar, often used as a preservative for foodstuffs and an intravenous nutrient

glucose: blood sugar; a product of the body's assimilation of carbohydrates, and a major source of energy

glutamic acid: an amino acid present in all complete proteins; usually manufactured from vegetable protein; used as a salt substitute and a flavor-intensifying agent

glutamine: an amino acid that constitutes, with glucose, the major nourishment used by the nervous system

GRAS: Generally Recognized As Safe; a list established by Congress to cover substances added to food

hesperidin: part of the C complex

holistic treatment: treatment of the whole person

hormone: a substance formed in endocrine organs and transported by body fluids to activate other specifically receptive organs

humectant: a substance that is used to preserve the moisture content of materials

hydrolyzed protein chelate: water soluble and chelated for easy assimilation

hydrolyzed: put into water-soluble form

hypervitaminosis: a condition caused by an excessive ingestion of vitamins

hypoglycemia: a condition caused by abnormally low blood sugar

hypovitaminosis: a deficiency disease due to an absence of vitamins in the diet

immune: protected against disease

insulin: the hormone, secreted by the pancreas, concerned with the metabolism of sugar in the body

IU: International Units

lactating: producing milk

laxative: a substance that stimulates evacuation of the bowels

linoleic acid: one of the polyunsaturated fats, a constituent of lecithin; known as vitamin F; indispensable for life, and must be obtained from foods

lipid: a fat or fatty substance

lipofuscin: age pigment in cells

lipotropic: preventing abnormal or excessive accumulation of fat in the liver

megavitamin therapy: treatment of illness with massive amounts of vitamins

metabolize: to undergo change by physical and chemical processes

nitrites: used as fixatives in cured meats; can combine with natural stomach and food chemicals to cause dangerous cancer-causing agents called nitroscimines

orthomolecular: the right molecule used for the right treatment; doctors who practice preventive medicine and use vitamin therapies are known as orthomolecular physicians

OSHA: Occupational Safety and Health Administration

oxalates: organic chemicals found in certain foods, especially spinach, which can combine with calcium to form calcium oxalate, an insoluble chemical the body cannot use

PABA: para-amniobenzoic acid; a member of the B complex

palmitate: water-solublized vitamin A

polyunsaturated fats: highly nonsaturated fats from vegetable sources; tend to lower blood cholesterol

predigested protein: protein that has been processed for fast assimilation and can go directly to the bloodstream

pro-vitamin: a vitamin precursor; a chemical substance necessary to produce a vitamin

PUFA: polyunsaturated fatty acid

RDA: Recommended Daily Dietary Allowances as established by the Food and Nutrition Board, National Academy of Sciences National Research Council

RNA: the abbreviation used for ribonucleic acid

rose hips: a rich source of vitamin C; the nodule underneath the bud of a rose called a hip, in which the plant produces the vitamin C we extract

rutin: a substance extracted from buckwheat; part of the C complex

saturated fatty acids: usually solid at room temperature; higher proportions found in foods from animal sources; tend to raise blood cholesterol levels

sequestrant: a substance that absorbs ions and prevents changes that would affect flavor, texture, and color of food; used for water softening

syncope: brief loss of consciousness; fainting

synergistic: the action of two or more substances to produce an effect that each alone could not accomplish

synthetic: produced artificially

teratological: monstrous or abnormal formations in animals or plants

tocopherols: the group of compounds (alpha, beta, delta, epsilon, eta, gamma, and zeta) that make vitamin E; obtained through vacuum distillation of edible vegetable oils

toxicity: the quality or condition of being poisonous, harmful, or destructive

toxin: an organic poison produced in living or dead organisms

triglycerides: fatty substances in the blood

unsaturated fatty acids: most often liquid at room temperature; primarily found in vegetable fats

USAN: United States Adopted Names Council; cosponsored by the American Pharmaceutical Association (APhA), the American Medical Association (AMA), and the United States Pharmacopia (USP) for the specific purpose of coining suitable, acceptable, nonproprietary names in the drug field

U.S. RDA: United States Recommended Daily Allowances

xerosis: a condition of dryness

zein: protein from corn

zyme: a fermenting substance

PART TWO
GETTING YOURS

XIV

Your Special Vitamin Needs

101. Selecting Your Regimen

We all know that not everyone has the same metabolism, but we often forget that this also means that not everyone requires the same vitamins. In the following sections I have outlined a number of personalized regimens for a variety of specialized needs. Look them all over and see which ones best fit your own special situation. If you fall under more than one category, adjust the combined regimens so that you are not double-dosing yourself, only adding the additional vitamins.

You will notice that in many cases I advise what I call an nsp, a nutrition starter program. This basic vitamin trio, taken twice daily, is my foundation for general good health.

- High-potency multiple vitamin with chelated minerals (time release preferred)
- Vitamin C, 1,000 mg. with bioflavonoids, rutin, hesperidin, and rose hips
- High-potency chelated multiple minerals, 1 of each with breakfast and dinner

Please note: Before starting any program you should check "Cautions" (section 98) and with a nutritionally oriented doctor—*the regimens in this book are not prescriptive nor are they intended as medical advice.*

102. Women

12–18   Multiple vitamin and mineral
Vitamin C, 500 mg. with rose hips
Vitamin E, 200 IU (dry form)
1 of each with breakfast

19–50   High-potency multiple vitamin and mineral (time release preferred)
Vitamin C, 1,000 mg, with bioflavonoids
Vitamin E, 400 IU (dry form)
1 of each with breakfast, and again with evening meal if necessary
Also, 3 RNA-DNA, 100-mg. tablets daily
1 multiple digestive enzyme when needed
Stress B complex A.M. and P.M. if stress conditions exist

50+   Multiple vitamin and mineral (time release preferred)
Vitamin C, 1,000 mg. with bioflavonoids
Vitamin E, 400 IU (dry form)

1 of each with breakfast; repeat at evening meal if desired
3 RNA-DNA 100-mg. tablets daily
2 multiple minerals daily
1–3 multiple digestive enzymes daily

103. Men

11–18   Multiple vitamin and mineral
        Vitamin C, 500 mg. with rose hips
        Vitamin E, 400 IU (dry form)
        1 of each with breakfast

19–50   High-potency multiple vitamin and mineral (time release preferred)
        Vitamin C, 1,000 mg. with bioflavonoids
        Vitamin E, 400 IU (dry form)
        1 of each A.M. and P.M.
        3 RNA-DNA 100-mg. tablets daily
        2 multiple minerals
        lecithin granules, 2 tbsp. or 9 capsules daily
        Stress B complex A.M. and P.M. if needed

50+   Multiple vitamin and mineral
        Vitamin C, 1,000 mg. with bioflavonoids
        Vitamin E, 400 IU (dry form)
        1 of each twice a day
        3 RNA-DNA 100-mg. tablets daily
        2 multiple minerals
        1–3 multiple digestive enzymes daily

104. Infants

1–4   One good-tasting chewable multiple vitamin daily (check label to see that

all the primary vitamins are included);
there should be no artificial color,
flavors, or sugar (sucrose) added.

105. Children

4–12   Growing children need a stronger multiple vitamin containing minerals, especially calcium and iron, for normal
growth. The tablet should also be high
in B complex and vitamin C (50 percent of American children do not even
get the RDA for vitamin C). One daily
is sufficient (check label to be sure
there is no artificial color, flavor, or
sugar [sucrose] added).

106. Pregnant Women

The right vitamins are essential at this time:

A good high-potency multiple vitamin and mineral rich in vitamins A, B_6, B_{12}, C, and folic
acid
Multiple chelated minerals, rich in calcium (2
tablets should equal 1,000 mg. calcium and
500 mg. magnesium)
1 of each twice daily
Also, folic acid, 800 mg. 3 times a day

107. Nursing Mothers

The same supplements recommended for pregnant women plus additional vitamins A, B_6, B_{12},

and C. Your body and your baby need the best nourishment you can give them.

108. Runners

During the first fifteen to twenty minutes of running you burn up almost only glucose. The body then comes in with fats (lipids) for energy (in utilizing lipids for energy, a compound called acetyl-coenzyme-A is formed). If there are only animal fats present, the compound forms slowly and energy is insufficient. If polyunsaturates are present, on the other hand, the compound forms quickly. Increase your intake of polyunsaturates—seeds, peanuts—and antioxidants, such as vitamin A, C, E, and selenium, to avoid free radical reactions.

A good supplement program would be:

Multiple vitamin with chelated minerals
Vitamin C complex, 1,000 mg.
Stress B complex
1 of each 2–3 times a day
Also, vitamin E, 400 IU A.M. and P.M. and 1
   multiple chelated mineral tablet daily

109. Joggers

The nutritional needs of joggers are the same as those for runners. Just remember: for highest energy keep polyunsaturates in mind.

With tension and stress an accepted part of your daily life, and energy a necessity, you need a vitamin regimen that won't let you down. Many high-level executives I know use this one:

nsp
Stress B complex A.M. and P.M.
Lecithin granules, 2 tbsp. or 3 capsules with each
  meal
B_{15}, 50 mg. 1–3 times daily

If you're in a hurry in the morning, you might want to try my high-energy breakfast drink:

RECIPE:

2 tbsp. protein powder
1 tbsp. natural yeast
2 tbsp. lecithin powder
3 ice cubes
2 tbsp. fresh fruit, honey, or fructose

Mix in blender at high speed for one minute.

111. Students.

Eating on the run, skipping breakfast, and not getting enough rest is a way of life for most students. And as if this isn't bad enough for good health, student diets usually consist of mostly starches and carbohydrates. If you're in this category, be aware that these factors, as well as your constant stress situations at school, are taking their toll. A good supplement program would be:

nsp
Vitamin E, 400 IU
Stress B complex
1 of each with breakfast and dinner

Also, you might improve your work performance by increasing your intake of choline-rich foods. (See section 35.)

112. Senior Citizens

The nutritional needs of senior citizens may vary widely, depending on the individual. As a general rule, however, if you're over sixty-five you need extra minerals, especially calcium, magnesium, and iron, as well as extra vitamins such as B complex and C. Vitamin E can help alleviate poor circulation, which is so often responsible for leg cramps. And don't forget about fiber. If chewing is a problem, high-fiber foods can be ground to convenient sizes or textures and are just as effective. Also, sweets should be discouraged, as there is a high incidence of sugar diabetes among older people.

A good supplement regimen would be:

Multiple vitamin and mineral
Rose hips vitamin C, 500 mg, with bioflavoids
Multiple chelated mineral tablet
Vitamin E, 400 IU (dry form)
1 of each with breakfast and dinner

113. Athletes

Athletes have very demanding nutritional needs. The prime nutritional requirements for performance is energy, and high-energy foods —as opposed to "quick-energy" foods—should be eaten. If you're involved in action sports, you need a diet with more carbohydrates and protein than someone involved in a low-energy sport. Then again, even golf can become a high-energy game when carried on intensively for a long time. Keep in mind that excess amounts of glucose, sugar, honey, or hard candy tend to draw fluid into the gastrointestinal tract. This can add to dehydration problems in endurance performance. A thirst-quenching tart drink of frozen or canned fruit juice is the best quick-energy beverage.

For supplements, I recommend:

Multiple vitamin and chelated minerals
Stress B complex
Vitamin C complex, 1000 mg.
Vitamin E, 400–1,000 IU
Multiple chelated minerals
1 of each with breakfast, lunch, and dinner

A protein supplement is also a good idea.

114. Night Workers

The Center for Research on Stress and Health at the Stanford Research Institute has found that "the rotating shift exacts a heavy physical and emotional toll from workers." When eating and sleeping patterns are disrupted, so are the body's biological rhythms, and it takes "three to four weeks for the circadian rhythms to become synchronized." If you change from day to night shifts often, your body is under much stress, your chances of illness are greater, and your risk of ulcers is high. I feel that supplements are essential:

nsp
1 vitamin D, 400 IU with largest meal
3 tryptophan tablets a half hour before bedtime
(whenever that happens to be)

115. Truck Drivers

Tension, stress, and a diet that is all too often high in greasy foods are important reasons for considering the following supplements:

nsp
Lecithin granules, 3 tbsp. or 12 capsules daily
1 B complex, 100 mg.
3 tryptophan tablets a half hour before bedtime
if needed for sleep

116. Dancers

Dancers have energy requirements that rank with those of athletes, but because of weight restrictions they cannot consume the same amount of carbohydrates. Good supplements are indispensable, as most dancers will tell you. I suggest:

nsp (be sure to take the multiple mineral twice daily)

1 balanced calcium and magnesium supplement daily

B$_{15}$, 50 mg. 3 times daily

117. Construction Workers

One out of every four workers is exposed to substances considered hazardous, according to the National Institute for Occupational Safety and Health (NIOSH). Construction workers are particularly vulnerable. Depending upon the sort of construction you're doing and where you're doing it, you're exposed to a variety of harmful conditions from general pollution to inhaling lead oxide, which can happen if you're soldering scrap metal or plastics. In any event, a diet rich in antioxidants such as vitamins A, C, and E will help detoxify your body. The following supplements are recommended:

nsp
B complex, 100 mg. twice daily
Vitamin E, 400–1,000 IU twice daily

118. Gamblers

If you're a gambler, I don't have to tell you about your stress, sleep, and dietary needs. I'm sure you're aware that all three are higher than average. What you might not realize, though, is that you could be in need of vitamin-D supplementation because of lack of sunlight. For best performance at any table, I suggest the following supplements:

214

nsp
Vitamin E, 400 IU twice daily
Vitamin D, 400 IU if necessary

119. Salespersons

The daily grind of having to deal with the public cannot be underestimated. Whether you're selling automobiles, books, exercise machines, or food, doing it on the road or from behind a counter, the emotional and physical stress on your body is great. And because appearances are often as important as products in your line of work, you'd be wise to pack the right supplements along with your samples. You'll be happily surprised with the results.

nsp
Stress B complex 3 times daily (with each meal)
Vitamin E, 400 IU A.M. and P.M.

120. Actors

There's not an actor or actress I know who doesn't need a B-vitamin supplement. The stress and tension of performance is an occupational given. And if you're like most theatrical performers, dieting is the only form of eating you know, too often denying you necessary vitamins. A helpful supplement scenario would be:

nsp
Stress B complex A.M. and P.M.
Vitamin E, 400 IU twice daily

121. Singers

Like actors, singers are also under high levels of stress, whether performing or rehearsing. If you worry about laryngitis, or other throat infections, it's advisable to keep your vitamin-C levels high at all times. Time-release vitamin C is your best choice.

nsp
Additional vitamim C, 1,000 mg. A.M. and P.M. when necessary

122. Doctors and Nurses

If you work with illness, you need all the protection you can get. Long hours, stress, and germs themselves, all contribute to your need for vitamin and mineral supplementation.

nsp
Stress B complex twice daily
Extra vitamin C to ward off infections

123. Handicapped

If you're disabled, your needs for vitamins are usually increased. More often than not, if one part of your body is not functioning properly, another part is working twice as hard—and needs nourishment. Helpful basic supplements would be:

1 B complex, 50 mg. A.M. and P.M.
1 high-potency multiple mineral twice daily

124. Golfers

As much as you enjoy it, golfing takes a lot out of you. The stress and tension of the game can use up B vitamins at a rapid clip. The right supplements might not get you down into the seventies, but they can help you stay energetic throughout the game.

nsp
Stress B complex A.M. and P.M.

125. Tennis Players

If you play tennis often, you might look good on the outside, but be a nutritional mess inside. I've found that far too many tennis buffs skip meals, or eat only protein—both bad habits. A demanding game like tennis requires that you serve yourself all the vitamins you need.

nsp
Stress B complex A.M. and P.M.
Extra calcium to prevent muscle fatigue
Vitamin B_{15}, 50 mg. 1–3 times daily
Vitamin E, 400–1,000 IU daily
Wheat-germ oil
Liver-yeast supplement

126. Teachers

School days are as stressful for teachers as they are for students, if not more so. To keep your energy and spirits up, a good vitamin program is important.

Stress B complex twice daily

127. Smokers

Every cigarette you smoke destroys about 25 mg. of vitamin C. Also, lung cancer risk aside, you're more prone to cardiovascular and pulmonary disorders than nonsmokers. Without going into the long list of deleterious effects cigarettes can have, I feel confident in telling smokers that they need all the nutritional help they can get, especially from antioxidants such as vitamins A, C, E, and selenium.

nsp
Vitamin C, 2,000 mg. A.M. and P.M.
Vitamin E, 400—1,000 IU daily
Selenium, 50 mcg. 1—3 times daily
Vitamin A, 10,000 IU daily

128. Drinkers

Alcoholism is the chief cause of vitamin deficiency among civilized people with ample food supplies. If you're a heavy drinker, the alcohol you consume usually takes the place of needed protein, or, in some cases, prevents absorption or proper storage of ingested vitamins.

nsp
B complex, 100 mg. twice daily (especially needed are B_1 B_6, and folic acid)

129. Excessive TV Watchers

Just because you spend a lot of time relaxing in front of your set doesn't mean you're not in need of extra vitamins. For the eyestrain it's more than likely that you need additional vitamin A. And if you rarely get to see the light of day, you might need vitamin D also.

nsp
Vitamin A, 10,000 IU with breakfast
Vitamin D, 400 IU 5 days a week if necessary

XV

The Right Vitamin at the Right Time

130. Special Situation Supplements

Your body's vitamin needs are not always the same and special situations require special food regimens and supplements. What follows is a list of such situations, most of them temporary, with supplement suggestions. For foods that offer specific vitamins and minerals see sections 24 through 65. Once again, this information is not prescriptive. (See section 101 for nsp.)

131. Acne

This scourge of teenage years has been treated in a variety of ways, from X-rays to tetracycline, with only varying degrees of success. I encourage more natural treatment of the condition, and have been delighted by the results.

Multiple vitamin *without* minerals, 1 daily
Vitamin E, 400 IU (dry form), 1–2 daily
Vitamin A, 25,000 IU (water soluble), 1–2 daily, 6 days a week
Zinc, 50 mg. chelated, 1 tablet 3 times daily with meals
Acidophilus liquid, 1–2 tbsp. 3 times daily, or 3–6 capsules 3 times daily

132. Athlete's Foot

Vitamin-C powder or crystals applied directly to the affected areas seems to help this fungus infection. Keep your feet dry, and out of shoes as much as possible, until the infection clears.

133. Bad Breath

Along with proper brushing and flossing, you might try:

nsp
1 chlorophyll tablet or capsule 1–3 times daily
3 acidophilus capsules 3 times daily, or 1–2 tbsp. flavored acidophilus
Zinc, 50 mg. 1–3 times daily

134. Baldness or Falling Hair

There are no guarantees, but many people report a definite diminution of hair loss with this regimen:

Stress B complex twice daily
Choline and inositol, 1,000 mg. of each daily
Daily jojoba oil scalp massage and shampoo
A multiple-mineral formula with 1,000 mg. calcium and 500 mg. magnesium, 1 daily

135. Bee Stings

The best thing to do about bee stings is to try to avoid them. Vitamin B_1 (thiamine) has been shown to be a fairly good insect repellent. Taken three times, daily, 100 mg. B_1 creates a smell at the level of your skin that insects do not like. If you're too late with the B_1 and do get stung, 1,000 mg. vitamin C could help ease the allergic reactions.

136. Bleeding Gums

The most effective vitamin therapy for bleeding gums is 1,000 mg. vitamin C complex, with bioflavonoids, rutin, and hesperidin, taken three times a day.

137. Broken Bones

If you've ever broken a bone, you know how frustrating it is waiting for it to mend. That feeling can be alleviated, and bone healing accelerated, by increasing your calcium and vitamin-D intakes. Daily doses of 1,000 mg. calcium and 400 IU vitamin D are good, or bonemeal tablets with vitamin D, 5 to 10 daily, would be equally effective.

138. Bruises

Vitamin C complex, 1,000 mg. with bioflavonoids, rutin, and hesperidin, taken three times
daily will help prevent capillary fragility, those
black-and-blue marks that occur when the tiny
blood vessels beneath the skin rupture.

139. Burns

The most important thing to do with a burn is
to put cold water on it immediately. To effectively stimulate wound healing, 50 mg. zinc
daily has been found useful and is worth trying.
Vitamin C complex, 1,000 mg. with bioflavonoids, taken in the morning and evening is recommended to prevent infections. Vitamin E,
1,000 IU used orally and topically can help
prevent scarring.

140. Cold Feet

If you're embarrassed by wearing socks to bed
all the time, you could try a good multimineral
supplement with iodine twice a day, along with
kelp tablets. The cold feet could be due to the
fact that your thyroid glands are not producing
enough thyroxin.

141. Cold Sores

Few things are more annoying than cold sores.
The best supplement remedy I've discovered is:

Vitamin C complex, 1,000 mg. with bioflavonoids A.M. and P.M.

Lactobacilus acidophilus, 3 capsules 3 times a
  day
Vitamin-E oil, 28,000 IU applied directly to
  affected area

142. Constipation

Everyone is bothered by constipation at some
time or other. Usually this is due to a lack of
bulk in the diet or because of certain medications, such as codine. Harsh laxatives can rob
the body of nutrients, as well as cause rebound
constipation and laxative dependency, so natural
remedies should be your first choice.

2 tbsp. unprocessed bran flakes daily
3–9 bran tablets daily
1 tbsp. acidophilus liquid 3 times daily
A vegetable laxative and stool softener for a
  short time if necessary

143. Cuts

Vitamin C complex, 1,000 mg. with bioflavonoids
twice daily, along with 50 mg. zinc and 1,000 IU
vitamin E.

144. Dry Skin

Vitamin-E oil seems to work wonders when
applied to dry skin, as do oils rich in vitamin A
and vitamin D. As a dietary supplement, if
you're not eating enough sweet potatoes, carrots, liver, and tomatoes, try 25,000 IU vitamin
A daily for two weeks, then cut dosage back
to 10,000 IU. If you've cut all fats from your

diet, put some back in the form of polyunsaturated oil. Two tablespoons on your daily salad is ample. Or try 3 to 6 lecithin capsules three times daily, along with nsp.

145. Hangovers

To prevent them, take 1 B complex, 100 mg., before going out, 1 again while you're drinking, and another right before going to bed. (Alcohol destroys B complex.)

If you already have one, take 1 B complex, 100 mg., three times daily. Portable oxygen works wonders.

146. Hay Fever

Stress can cause hay fever attacks to worsen. If you're one of the many who suffer, you might find relief with 1 stress B complex twice daily, pantothenic acid, 100 mg. three times daily, and extra vitamin C, which has evidenced effective antihistamine properties.

147. Headaches

A surprisingly effective vitamin-mineral regimen for headaches is:

100 mg. niacin 3 times daily

100 mg. stress B complex (time release) twice daily

Calcium and magnesium (twice as much calcium as magnesium is the proper ratio), which are nature's tranquilizers

148. Heartburn

Over-the-counter antacids, such as Gelusil, Winger, Kolantyl, Maalox, Di-Gel, Rolaids, contain aluminum, which disturbs calcium and phosphorus metabolism. You'll probably be better off taking 5 bonemeal tablets daily (with food), multiple digestive enzymes one to three times daily, and drinking fluids before or after meals, *not* during.

149. Hemorrhoids

Just about half the people over fifty are afflicted by hemorrhoids. Improper diet, lack of exercise, and straining at stool are all contributing factors. And coffee, chocolate, cola, and cocoa are accessories to the discomfort by promoting anal itching. If you're bothered by hemorrhoids, 1 tablespoon of unprocessed bran three times a day is helpful, along with 1,000 mg. vitamin C complex twice a day for healing membranes, and 3 acidophilus capsules three times a day (or 1 to 2 tablespoons of acidophilus liquid one to three times a day).

150. Insomnia

Barbiturates, such as phenobarbital, Seconal, Nembutal, and Butisol, are strong sedatives and hypnotics that are two often prescribed for insomnia. Aside from being habit forming and dangerous if mixed with other drugs, these barbiturates can also cause low calcium levels.

Tryptophan, on the other hand, is a natural

amino acid that is essential to our bodies, and which, according to recent research at the Maryland Psychiatric Research Center, induces sleep.

An effective insomnia program:

3 tryptophan tablets a half hour before bedtime
1 chelated calcium and magnesium tablet 3 times daily and 3 tablets a half hour before bedtime

Milk, as you know, is a fine natural source of calcium, and turkey is a good source of tryptophan. An open-face turkey sandwich and a glass of warm milk before bedtime could be the sleep remedy of your life.

151. Itching

As an antihistamine, 2 1,000-mg. vitamin-C tablets (time release) in the morning and in the evening, with food, might be helpful. I would also recommend a stress B complex with breakfast and dinner, 100 mg. pantothenic acid one to three times daily, and vitamin-E cream applied to afflicted area three times daily.

152. Jet Lag

So your plane from London lands at 9 A.M. and you're supposed to be at a meeting at 10 A.M. No problem, except for the fact that as far as your body is concerned, it's still only 4 A.M. and you should be asleep. Your best bet is to help your system catch up with your schedule by giving it the vitamins it needs.

227

Stress B complex (time release) A.M. and P.M. (start while on the plane).

nsp
Vitamin E, 400 IU twice daily

If you're feeling run-down, as well as tired, be sure to take additional vitamin C.

153. Leg Pains

Increase your calcium. Try 1 chelated calcium and magnesium tablet with breakfast and dinner, along with a chelated multiple mineral. Vitamin E has been reported quite helpful in cases of charley horse. The most common doses for it are 400 to 1,000 IU vitamin E one to three times daily.

154. Menopause

Because of the risks that have recently been brought to light about estrogens, many women have been seeking other ways to relieve the discomforts of menopause. A good number of menopausal women have found that 400 IU vitamin E one to three times a day does indeed alleviate hot flashes. If you're at that time of life, nsp and a 600-mg. stress B complex twice a day also seem to help.

155. Menstruation

Between the cramps and the bloating, menstruation is for most women a monthly annoyance. But this annoyance can dwindle down to a mere distraction once the discomfort is alleviated.

Vitamin B$_6$, 50 mg. 3 times daily (most effective as a natural diuretic)
B complex, 100 mg. (time release) A.M. and P.M.
nsp

156. Motion Sickness

This is one condition where remedies are most effective if taken beforehand. Vitamins B$_1$ and B$_6$ are the nutrients of choice (in fact, many prenatal antinausea preparations contain vitamin B$_6$). Taking 100 mg. B complex the night before you leave and the morning of your trip has been found to be effective by many queasy travelers.

157. Muscle Soreness

For that ache-all-over feeling after a workout, or just general muscle soreness, I've seen many people find relief with vitamin E, 400 to 1,000 IU taken one to three times daily. A chelated multiple mineral in the morning and at night also has helped.

158. The Pill

If you take oral contraceptives, not only are you more vulnerable than other women to blood clots, strokes, and heart attacks, but you're also more likely to be deficient in zinc, folic acid, vitamins, C, B$_6$, and B$_{12}$ (which accounts for much nervousness and depression among pill takers).

Supplements are important:

nsp
Zinc, 50 mg. chelated, 1–3 tablets daily
Folic acid, 800 mcg. 1–3 times daily
B_{12}, 2,000 mg. (time release), A.M.
B_6, 50 mg. 1–3 times daily

159. Poison Ivy

Vitamin-E oil or aloe vera gel applied externally can help healing. Two 1,000 mg. vitamin C complex (time release) taken A.M. and P.M. along with vitamin E, 400 to 1,000 IU should alleviate the itching.

160. Polyps

These small annoying growths should definitely be seen by a doctor, and in most instances surgical removal is necessary. But as far as supplements go, Dr. Jerome J. DeCosse, professor and chairman of surgery at the Medical College of Wisconsin, used 3,000 mg. vitamin C (time release) daily on patients with polyps, and had noteworthy success with the treatment.

161. Postoperative Healing

After surgery, your body needs all the nutritional support it can get.

Vitamin E, 400 IU (dry form), 3 times daily

2 vitamin C complex, 1,000 mg. with bioflavonoids, hesperidin, and rutin A.M. and P.M.

High-potency multiple vitamin with chelated minerals A.M. and P.M.

High-potency multiple chelated mineral tablet A.M. and P.M.

Vitamin A, 10,000–25,000 IU 3 times daily for 5 days (stop for 2 days to prevent build up)

162. Prickly Heat

Much like itching, prickly heat seems to respond to the antihistamine properties of vitamin C. (See section 123 for regimen.)

163. Prostate Problems

Chronic prostitis, where inflammation of the gland is the case as opposed to infection, has been found to respond to treatment with zinc. (The prostate gland normally contains about ten times more zinc than any other organ in the body.) In many cases, symptoms have completely disappeared.

nsp

Zinc, 50 mg. 3 times daily

Vitamin F or lecithin capsules (1200 mg.), 3 caps 3 times daily

164. Psoriasis

Though many jokes have been made about this disease, it is no laughing matter to the millions who suffer from it. No one treatment has been found to be totally effective, but the following has met with much success:

nsp

Vitamin A (water soluble), 10,000 IU 3 times daily for 6 days a week

B complex, 100 mg. (time released) A.M. and P.M.

Rose hips vitamin C, 1,000 mg. A.M. and P.M. (this is in addition to the vitamin C called for in the nsp)

Vitamin E (dry form), 400 IU 3 times daily

3 vitamin-F for lecithin capsules 3 times daily

Increase protein (preferably animal source)

165. Stopping Smoking

It's no mean feat to stop smoking, and your body knows it. Those withdrawal symptoms are real. For the irritability that occurs, 1 tryptophan (667 mg.) tablet three times a day seems to help. Also 1 B complex, 100 mg. (time release), taken with the evening meal. Don't forget the nsp.

166. Sunburn

A good sunscreening preparation should always be used before exposing yourself to the sun's ultraviolet rays for any length of time. What most people don't realize is that the sun actually burns the skin, and bad burns can break the skin and leave it vulnerable to infection.

If it's too late for preventives, try this:

Aloe vera gel applied 3–4 times daily

A PABA cream or vitamin-E cream (20,000 IU) also applied 3–4 times daily

nsp
Additional vitamin C, 1,000 mg. A.M. and P.M.
until burn heals

167. Teeth Grinding

People are usually unaware of grinding their
teeth. It occurs more often in children than
adults, and most often during sleep. Nsp; B complex, 100 mg. A.M. and P.M.; and a few bonemeal tablets nightly before sleep can help.

168. Varicose Veins

Age, lack of exercise, and chronic constipation
are contributing factors to varicose veins. Watch-
ing your diet and exercising regularly can do a
lot toward preventing them. Nsp with an extra
1,000 mg. vitamin C complex twice daily has
been found to help, along with 400 to 800 IU
vitamin E.

169. Vasectomy

Men with vasectomies are more susceptible to
infections and would be wise to take an additional 1,000 mg. vitamin C complex daily,
along with regular nsp diet supplementation.

170. Warts

They don't come from handling frogs, but they
do seem to effectively disappear when treated
with vitamin-E oil. The most successful regimen

appears to be 28,000 IU vitamin E applied externally one to two times daily and 400 IU vitamin E (dry form) taken internally three times a day.

XVI

Getting Well and Staying That Way

171. Why You Need Supplements During Illness

During illness the body is under stress. Cells are destroyed, exhausted adrenal glands deprived of nutrients are unable to function properly, and the body's stress-fighting team of vitamin C, B₆, folic acid, and pantothenic acid is severely depleted.

Because we require these vitamins to effectively utilize other nutrients and to keep our metabolism functioning all the time, our need for them is obviously increased when we're ill. And since we know that fever and stress rob our body of its most essential nutrients, the importance of supplements is self-evident.

Again, the following regimens are not in-

tended as medical advice, only as a guide in
working with your doctor.

172. Allergies

Allergies come in all shapes and sizes, with all
sorts of symptoms, and you can contact them
for just about anything. Nonetheless, they take
their nutritional toll, and supplements can help.

1 stress B complex with vitamin C 3 times daily
Pantothenic acid, 100 mg. 3 times daily
nsp

If you have an allergy, it would be a good
idea to take a hard look at your present diet.
Many allergies are caused by MSG, food color-
ing, additives, and preservatives.

173. Arthritis

Thousands upon thousands of people suffer from
this painful chronic condition. Because it puts
so much stress on the body, vitamin-mineral
supplementation is really essential.

nsp
Extra vitamin C, 1,000 mg. 1–3 times a day (if
  you take a lot of aspirin, you're losing vitamin
  C)
B complex, 100 mg. 1–3 times a day
B12, up to 2,000 mcg. daily
Niacin up to 1 g. daily
1–3 yucca tabs 3 times daily
Pantothenic acid, 100 mg. 3 times daily
Vitamin A, 10,000 IU, and vitamin D, 400 IU,

1–3 capsules 3 times daily (take for 5 days and stop for 2)

or

Cod liver oil, 1–2 tbsp. 3 times daily (if capsules, 3 caps 3 times daily). Again, take for 5 days and stop for 2

174. Blood Pressure—High and Low

High: Lecithin granules, 3 tbsp. daily or 3 caps 3 times daily. Potassium may be necessary if you are taking an antihypertensive

nsp

Vitamin E, 100 IU daily and work up to higher strengths (check with your doctor)

Low: 1–3 kelp tablets daily

nsp

175. Bronchitis

This inflammation of the bronchial tube lining is quite common and extremely enervating. The stress it puts on the body is high, and even antibiotics are the bad guys as far as nutrients are concerned. (See section 206.)

Vitamin A, 25,000 IU 1–3 times daily (take for 5 days then stop for 2)

Rose hips vitamin C, 1,000 mg. A.M. and P.M.

nsp

Vitamin E, 400 IU (dry form) 1–3 times daily

Water, 6–8 glasses daily

3 acidophilus caps 3 times daily or 1–2 tbsp.
liquid 3 times daily

176. Chicken Pox

This childhood staple is caused by a virus closely
related to that of shingles. The fever and itching
deplete a good amount of nutrients. Many moth-
ers have found their children up and about
faster by adding the following supplements to
their diets.

Rose hips vitamin C, 500 mg. 3 times daily
Vitamin E, 100–200 IU 1–3 times daily
Vitamin A, 10,000 IU daily (check pediatrician
for proper dosage according to age and
weight). Take for 5 days and stop for 2
Multivitamin and mineral A.M. and P.M.

177. Colds

No one pays too much attention to a cold, except
the body it pays plenty.
nsp
Rose hips vitamin C, 1,000 mg. 3 times daily
Vitamin A, 25,000 IU 1–3 times daily (take for
5 days and stop for 2)
Vitamin E, 400 IU (dry form) 1–3 times daily
Water, 6–8 glasses daily
3 acidophilus capsules 3 times daily or 1–2 tbsp.
liquid 3 times daily

178. Colitis

As a rule this illness is more common in women
than men and often triggered by emotional up-

set. Alternating diarrhea and constipation, as well as abdominal pain, are its distressing hallmarks. Diet is of prime importance and vitamins are recommended.

nsp

Potassium, 99 mg. (elemental) 1–3 times daily

Sugarless cabbage juice (vitamin U), 1 glass 3 times daily

Water, 6–8 glasses daily

Aloe vera gel (for internal use), 1 tbsp. 3 times daily or 1–3 capsules 3 times daily

3–6 acidophilus caps 3 times daily or 2 tbsp. liquid 3 times daily

1 tbsp. bran flakes 3 times daily or 3–6 bran tablets

179. Diabetes

What happens in diabetes, primarily, is that the pancreas fails to produce adequate insulin and the blood sugar rises uncontrollably. In mild cases diet alone can control the condition. (Beware of hidden sugars. See section 231.) In severe cases, replacement insulin is necessary. In all cases, the care of a physician is essential.

Supplements that have aided diabetics are:

nsp

Chromium, 1–2 mg. daily for 6 months

Potassium, 99 mg. 3 times daily

Chelated zinc, 50 mg. 1–3 times daily

Water, 6–8 glasses daily

180. Eye Problems

From simple inflammations to refraction difficulties to serious diseases, eye problems should never be ignored, nor should visits to the ophthalmologist or optometrist be postponed. There are, however, generally beneficial supplements you can take.

Vitamin A, 10,000 IU 1–3 times daily (take for 5 days, then stop for 2)
B complex, 100 mg. (time release) A.M. and P.M.
Rose hips vitamin C complex, 500 mg. A.M. and P.M.
Vitamin E, 400 IU (dry form) A.M. and P.M.

181. Heart Conditions

With any heart condition, you should be under a doctor's care. Though the following supplements have been found to be quite safe and helpful, you should check with your physician to make sure they are not contraindicated in your particular case. (Vitamin E can increase the imbalance between the two sides of the heart for some people with rheumatic hearts.)

Vitamin B, 100 mg. (time release) A.M. and P.M.
Extra niacin, 100 mg. 1–3 times daily
Vitamin E, 400 IU (dry form), 1 daily
nsp
3 lecithin capsules or 3 tbsp. granules 3 times daily.

182. Hypoglycemia

Though an estimated 20 to 40 million Americans have it, this disease is one of the most often undiagnosed. It is a condition of low blood sugar, and, like diabetes, presents a situation where the body is unable to metabolize carbohydrates normally. Since a hypoglycemic's system overreacts to sugar, producing too much insulin, the key to raising blood sugar levels is not by eating rapidly metabolized carbohydrates but by eating more protein. (See section 232 for a balanced program.)

Recommended supplements:

Vitamin A and D capsules (10,000 and 400 IU 1–3 times daily for 5 days, then stop for 2

Vitamin C, 500 mg. with or after each meal

Vitamin E, 100–200 IU 3 times daily

B complex, 50 mg. 3 times daily

Vitamin F 1 capsule 3 times daily

Multiple mineral tab A.M. and P.M. (Niacin as needed and tolerated. See section 42.)

Pantothenic acid, 200 mg. 3 times daily

2 lecithin capsules (9 grains = 1,200 mg.) 3 times daily

Digestive enzymes if necessary

1 kelp tablet 3 times daily

3 acidophilus capsules or 1–2 tbsp. liquid 3 times daily

183. Impetigo

Caused by germs similar to those that cause boils—staphylococcus or streptococcus—it occurs more in children than adults, but no one is immune. It often results from scratching and infecting insect bites, allowing the germs to get into broken skin.

Vitamin A and D capsules (10,000 and 400 IU) 1–3 times daily (reduce dose for child) for 5 days, then stop for 2
Vitamin E, 100–400 IU (dry form) once a day
Rose hips vitamin C, 500 mg. A.M. and P.M.

184. Measles

You can get measles at any age, though it's more common among children. It is the most contagious of the communicable diseases. There is now a preventive vaccine for it, but the virus still manages to get a large number of the unprotected each year. The disease and rash can be mild, or severe with a heavy cough. Your body needs vitamins to help fight and recover from it.

Vitamin A, 10,000 IU (reduce dose for child) 1–3 times daily for 5 days, then stop for 2
Rose hips vitamin C, 500–1,000 mg. A.M. and P.M.
Vitamin E, 200–400 IU (dry form) A.M. *or* P.M.

185. Mononucleosis

Commonly contracted by adolescents and young adults, mono (glandular fever) or "the kissing disease" as it is often called, can happen to anyone and can deplete the body of massive amounts of nutrients.

Diet is important and supplements are generally considered essential during the long convalescence.

nsp
Extra vitamin C, 1,000 mg. A.M. and P.M. for 3 months
Potassium, 99 mg. 3 times daily
B complex, 100 mg. (time release) A.M. and P.M.

186. Mumps

A vaccine for mumps exists, but the disease is still quite common and just as nutritionally debilitating. The virus can spread through the patient's entire system, involving not only the salivary glands but the testicles or ovaries, the pancreas, the nervous system, and sometimes even the heart.

Vitamin A, 10,000 IU (reduce dose for children) 1–3 times daily for 5 days, then stop for 2
Rose hips vitamin C, 500–1,000 mg. twice daily
Vitamin E, 200–400 IU (dry form) daily

187. Shingles

Shingles (herpes zoster) is caused by a virus much like the one that causes chicken pox. But where chicken pox causes a general skin eruption, shingles usually erupts along a nerve path. Differences aside, the nutritional deficit caused by both diseases is high.
Vitamin A, 10,000–25,000 IU 1–3 times daily for 5 days, then stop for 2

Vitamin B complex, 100 mg. (time release) A.M. and P.M.

Rose hips vitamin C with bioflavonoids, 1,000–2,000 mg. A.M. and P.M.

Vitamin D, 1,000 IU 1–3 times daily for 5 days, then stop for 2

188. Tonsillitis

An inflammation of the tonsils that can afflict any age group, though it is more common in children. Good nutrition and supplements have been effective in preventing it as well as recovering from it.

nsp

Vitamin A, 10,000–25,000 IU (reduce dose for children) 1–3 times daily for 5 days, then stop for 2

Extra vitamin C complex, 1,000 mg. A.M. and P.M.

Vitamin E, 400 IU (dry form) 1–3 times daily

3 acidophilus caps or 1–2 tbsp. 3 times daily

Water, 6–8 glasses daily

189. Ulcers

There are two types of peptic ulcer, one in the stomach and the other in the duodenum, usually associated with excessive acidity in the stomach juices. (See section 9.) For both of these conditions, supplements have been found helpful.

Vitamin A, 25,000 IU 1–3 times daily for 5 days, then stop for 2

Vitamin B complex, 100 mg. (time release) A.M.
and P.M.
Rose hips vitamin C with bioflavonoids, 1,000
mg. (time release) A.M. and P.M.
High-potency multiple mineral A.M. and P.M.
Aloe vera gel, 1–3 capsules or 1–3 tbsp. liquid
daily

190. Venereal Disease

Syphilis and gonorrhea are the main types of
venereal disease. Sulfa drugs, penicillin, tetracycline, erythromycin, and the newer antibiotics are the most effective treatments for
them, but these remedies cause almost as much
need for supplements as the diseases themselves.

nsp
3 acidophilus capsules or 1–2 tbsp. liquid 3 times
daily
Extra rose hips vitamin C, 1,000 mg. A.M. and
P.M.
Vitamin K, 100 mcg. daily if on extended antibiotic program

XVII

It's Not All in Your Mind

191. How Vitamins and Minerals Affect Your Moods

The first scientifically documented discovery to relate mental illness to diet occurred when it was found that pellagra (with its depression, diarrhea, and dementia) could be cured with niacin. After that, it was shown that supplementation with the whole B complex produced greater benefits than niacin alone.

Evidence of biochemical causes for mental disturbances continues to mount. Experiments have shown that symptoms of mental illness can be switched off and on by altering vitamin levels in the body.

> Even normal, happy people can become
> depressed when made deficient in
> niacin or folic acid.

Dr. R. Shulman, reporting in the *British Journal of Psychiatry*, found that forty-eight out of fifty-nine psychiatric patients had folic-acid deficiencies. Other research has shown that the majority of the mentally and emotionally ill are deficient in one or more of the B-complex vitamins or vitamin C. And even normal, happy people have been found to become depressed and experience other symptoms of emotional disturbance when made niacin or folic-acid deficient.

At California's Stanford University, Dr. Linus Pauling conducted a series of tests to determine individual vitamin needs. As part of the series, he administered massive doses of vitamin C (as much as 40 g.) to schizophrenics and discovered that little or none of it was discarded in the urine. Since the body expels what it doesn't need of the water-soluble vitamins, the test clearly indicated that the mentally ill needed more vitamin C—more than one thousand times the RDA—than the rest of us.

192. Vitamins and Minerals for Depression and Anxiety

The following vitamins and minerals have in many cases been found to be effective in the treatment of depression and anxiety.

Vitamin B_1 (thiamine)—large amounts appear to energize depressed people and tranquilize anxious ones

Vitamin B_6 (pyridoxine)—important for the function of the adrenal cortex

Pantothenic acid—has a tension-relieving effect.

Vitamin C (ascorbic acid)—essential for combatting stress

Vitamin E (alpha-tocopherol)—aids brain cells in getting their needed oxygen

Zinc—oversees body processes and aids in brain function

Magnesium—necessary for nerve functioning, known as the antistress mineral

Calcium—makes you less jumpy, more relaxed

193. Other Drugs Can Add to Your Problems

Alcohol is a nerve depressant. If you take tranquilizers and a drink, the combination of the two can cause a severe depression—or even death.

If you take Darvon with a tranquilizer, you might find yourself experiencing tremors and mental confusion. The same thing can happen if you combine a sedative with an antihistamine (such as any found in over-the-counter cold preparations).

Oral contraceptives deplete the body of B_6, B_{12}, folic acid, and vitamin C. If you're on the pill and depressed, it is not surprising. Your need for B^2, necessary for normal tryptophan metabolism, is fifty to a hundred times a non-pill-user's requirement.

XVIII

Environmental Pollution and You

194. The Worst Things in Life Are Free

You still have some control over the food you eat and the water you drink, but you're stuck with the air you breathe. And if you live in any major urban area today, you're breathing polluted air.

> Every year 200 million tons of potentially dangerous pollutants are released into the atmosphere.

With each breath you subject your lungs and body to a wide range of pollutants. No part of you is immune. Pollutants affect your nose, eyes, throat, skin, and internal organs as well.

In fact, it has been estimated that breathing air in the Los Angeles basin is equivalent to smoking a pack of cigarettes a day. And since each cigarette is estimated to cut twelve minutes off your life, every breath you take in a polluted environment brings you that much closer to where you don't want to go.

Every year 200 million tons of potentially dangerous pollutants are released into the atmosphere. From industrial processes, incinerators, automobiles, fossil-fuel-burning operations, electric power plants, refineries, and more, we are inundated with dust, smoke, fumes, gasses, and tiny particles of solid matter such as tars and poisonous heavy metals. And in one breath you can take in 70,000 such solid particles!

How does your body hold up against this kind of assault? Well, vitamins are your first line of defense. Especially the antioxidants— vitamins A, C, E, and selenium. These nutrients are capable of protecting other substances from oxidation. In other words, the free radicals (uncontrolled oxidations that damage cells) that are formed when we inhale pollutants are kept in check.

195. Know Your Antioxidants

Vitamin A protects mucous membranes of mouth, nose, throat, and lungs. It also helps protect vitamin C from oxidation, which allows your C to work better.

Vitamin C fights bacterial infections and reduces the effects of allergy-producing substances. It also protects vitamins A, E, and some of the B complex from oxidation.

Vitamin E protects vitamins B and C from oxidation. It has the ability to unite with oxygen and prevent it from being converted into toxic peroxides. It acts as an antipollutant for the lungs.

Selenium and vitamin E must both be present to correct a deficiency in either. The levels of selenium in the blood of people in various cities has been found to bear a direct relationship to cancer mortality. The higher the levels of selenium, the lower the cancer death rate—and vice versa.

196. On-the-Job Dangers

The National Institute for Occupational Safety and Health (NIOSH) estimates that one out of every four workers is exposed to substances that are considered hazardous.

The following is a list of work-related risks you might not know that you're taking:

Electrical engineers, electricians, and printers Exposure to electronic devices, fluorescent lights, disinfectants, measuring devices, or certain dyes and inks may subject you to an odorless mercury that can cause emotional disorders or even death.

Secretaries and receptionists Certain duplicating machines give off fumes that may cause visual problems, fatigue, and headaches. Some switchboards can release ozone, a colorless vapor that may cause respiratory disorders.

Paperhangers There are wallpapers coated

251

with vinyl chloride, apparently carcinogenic, a chemical that can easily be inhaled.

Dentists, dental hygienists   The silver amalgam, often used for fillings, contains mercury and can give off vapors. The Institute for Occupational Safety estimates that there are unhealthy levels of mercury in one out of every ten dentists' offices.

Mechanics   If you work with machinery that is cleaned with solvents, you can inhale vapors that may be injurious to your health, causing skin inflammations as well as liver and kidney disturbances.

Asbestos workers   It is estimated that 45 percent of asbestos-insulation workers will die of some form of cancer. (Breathing in buildings where asbestos has been sprayed on steel beams and may flake off could be dangerous to anyone's health.)

Have you taken an antioxidant today?

PART THREE
VITAMINS VS. DRUGS

XIX
Caffeine

197. Effects of Caffeine on the Body

There are no doubts about it, caffeine is a powerful drug. That's right, *drug*. Chances are you're not just enjoying your daily coffees or colas, you're addicted to them.

Caffeine acts directly upon the central nervous system. It brings about an almost immediate sense of clearer thought and lessens fatigue. It also stimulates the release of stored sugar from the liver, which accounts for the "lift" coffee, cola, and chocolate (the caffeine big three) give. But these benefits may be far outweighed by the side effects.

• The release of stored sugar places heavy stress on the endocrine system.

- Heavy coffee drinkers often develop nervousness or become jittery.
- Coffee-drinking housewives demonstrated symptoms typical of drug withdrawal when switched to a decaffinated beverage.
- Dr John Minton, professor of surgery at Ohio State University and specialist in cancer oncology, has found that excessive intake of methylxanthines (active chemicals in caffeine) can cause benign breast disease and prostate problems.
- Many doctors consider caffeine a culprit in hypertensive heart disease.
- Dr. Phillip Cole, in the British medical journal *Lancet*, reported a strong relationship between coffee consumption and cancer of the bladder and the lower urinary tract.
- People who drink five cups of coffee daily have a 50 percent greater chance of having heart attacks than noncoffee drinkers, according to the British medical journal.
- The *Journal of the American Medical Association* reports a disease called caffeinism, with symptoms of appetite loss, weight loss, irritability, insomnia, feelings of flushing, chills, and sometimes a low fever.
- Scientists at John Hopkins University have shown that caffeine can interfere with DNA replication.
- The Center for Science in the Public Interest advises pregnant women to stay away from caffeine, since studies have shown that the amount contained in about four cups of coffee per day causes birth defects in test animals.
- High doses of caffeine will cause laboratory animals to go into convulsions and then die.

Caffeine can be highly toxic (the lethal dose estimated to be around 10 g.). New research shows that one quart of coffee consumed in three hours can destroy much of the body's thiamine.

198. You're Getting More Than You Think

The following table shows the amount of caffeine (in milligrams) consumed in specific beverages and drugs:

BEVERAGE	12-OUNCE CAN OR BOTTLE
Coca-Cola	64.7 mg.
Dr. Pepper	60.9 mg.
Mountain Dew	54.7 mg.
Diet Dr. Pepper	54.2 mg.
Tab	49.4 mg.
Pepsi-Cola	43.1 mg.
R.C. Cola	33.7 mg.
Diet R.C.	33.0 mg.
Diet-Rite	31.7 mg.

Coffee	*Per Serving*
Instant	66.0 mg.
Percolated	110.0 mg.
Dripolated	146.0 mg.

Tea Bags	
Black 5-minute brew	46.0 mg.
Black 1-minute brew	28.0 mg.

Loose Tea	
Black 5-minute brew	40.0 mg.
Green 5-minute brew	35.0 mg.
Cocoa	13.0 mg.

DRUGS	PER PILL
Anacin	32.0 mg.
Cafergot	100.0 mg.
Empirin	32.0 mg.
Emprazil	30.0 mg.

Drugs	Per Pill
Excedrin	65.0 mg.
(Excedrin PM has no caffeine, but does have an antihistamine.)	
Fiorinal	130.0 mg.
Midol	32.4 mg.
Soma Compound	32.0 mg.
Triaminicin	30.0 mg.
Vanquish	33.0 mg.

199. Caffeine Alternatives

Decaffeinated coffee is *not* the best solution to the caffeine problem. Trichlorethylene, which was first used to remove caffeine, was found to cause a high incidence of cancer in test animals. Though the manufacturers have switched to methylene chloride, which is safer, it, too, introduces the same carbon-to-chlorine bond into the body that is characteristic of so many toxic insecticides.

Ginseng can give you a
real lift.

Regular tea is not the answer either, since that has nearly as much caffeine. But herb teas can be quite invigorating, and most natural-food stores have a wide variety to choose from. Then, too, ginseng can give you a real lift, much like the one you get from caffeine, without the side effects.

Colas, diet or regular, have become as popular as coffee for those who enjoy the caffeine boost. Try substituting club soda or mineral water, or even a flavored soda if you must. You won't get the caffeine lift, but you'll be doing your body a big favor.

XX
Alcohol

200. What It Does to Your Body

Alcohol is the most widely used drug in our society, and because it is so available, most people don't think of it as a drug. But it is; and if misused, it can cause a lot of damage to your body.

• Alcohol is not a stimulant, but actually a sedative-depressant of the central nervous system.
• It is capable of rupturing veins.
• It does not warm you up, but causes you to feel colder by increasing perspiration and body heat loss.
• It destroys brain cells by causing the withdrawal of necessary water from them.
• It can deplete the body of vitamin B_1, B_2, B_6,

B$_{12}$, folic acid, vitamin C, vitamin K, zinc, magnesium, and potassium.
• Four drinks a day are capable of causing organ damage.
• It can hamper the liver's ability to process fat.

201. What You Drink and When You Drink It

Just because the alcohol content varies in different beverages, don't be fooled. It is true that beer has only about 4 percent alcohol, wine about 12 percent, and whiskey up to 50 percent; but a can of beer, a glass of wine, and a shot of whiskey all have virtually the identical inebriation potential. In other words, four cans of beer can get you just as tipsy as four shots of tequila.

> A Bloody Mary at breakfast is
> more harmful than a whiskey
> sour at dinner.

Surprisingly, what you drink doesn't matter nearly as much as *when* you drink it. Dr. John D. Palmer, of the University of Massachusetts, reports that the length of time alcohol remains circulating in your blood varies throughout the day. Which means, of course, the more time the alcohol spends in your blood, the more time it has to act on your brain cells. Between 2 A.M. and noon are the most vulnerable hours, while late afternoon to early evening are the least. A cocktail at dinner will be burned away 25 percent faster than a Bloody Mary at breakfast. Dr. Palmer has also found that the last drink of a party, consumed after midnight, is metabolized relatively more slowly than the ones that preceded it, and will produce a more lasting rise in blood alcohol.

202. Vitamins to Decrease Your Taste for Alcohol

> Heavy drinkers can break
> the habit.

Research at the University of Texas by Professor Roger Williams has shown that if alcoholic mice are fed nutritious, vitamin-enriched diets, they quickly lose their interest in alcohol. This seems to hold true for people, since heavy drinkers have been able to break the habit—and even lose interest—with the right diet and proper nutritional supplements. Vitamins A, D, E, C, and all the B vitamins—especially B_{12}, B_6, and B_1—along with dolomite, choline, inositol, niacin, and a very high-protein diet have brought about the best results. Dr. H. L. Newbold, of New York, who has worked with alcoholics, recommends building up to 5 glutamine capsules (200 mg.)—not glutamic acid—three times a day to control drinking, and working with a good nutritionally oriented doctor for the best all-around regimen. (See section 128.)

In experiments done by the Veterans' Administration, a supplement of tryptophan, given in larger concentrations than occur in a normal diet, has helped alcoholics achieve normal sleeping patterns by reducing or normalizing the fragmentation of dreaming (REM). Because serotonin, a natural tranquilizer substance in the brain has been shown to be reduced in alcoholism, tryptophan can help alcoholics stay dry by relieving some of the symptoms of alcohol-related body chemistry disorders.

XXI

You and Your Rx

203. Why Vitamins Have Come Under Government Attack

Sickness is big business in the United States. The medical establishment considers current therapy to be drugs, surgery, and analysis. Period. Vitamins are rarely used in treatment, and preventive medicine is still in its infancy.

The situation is changing, however, because the public wants health professionals who are knowledgeable about nutrition.

Vitamins are natural substances and therefore not under government control. Many doctors don't like this, because the availability of vitamins can lead to the public's experimenting on its own. Large drug corporations don't like it because the substances are not patentable, which means they can't make money from them. But if vitamins were dangerous, the FDA would remove them from the market.

Needing a prescription for vitamins
would be like needing a prescription
for a pound of steak.

A few years ago the government tried to pass a law making high-potency vitamins and minerals available by prescription only. The public was outraged. It would be like having to obtain a prescription for a pound of beef, twenty carrots, six chicken livers. A huge letter-writing campaign was launched, and the bill was dropped. But many doctors and lots of drug companies would very much like to see it revived.

204. There Are Alternatives to Drugs

Americans consume over 1.5 million pounds of tranquilizers, more than 800,000 pounds of barbiturates, and well over 4 million pounds of antibiotics a year. Are all these drugs necessary? Probably not; but when people pay for a visit to their doctor, they expect to walk away with a prescription.

But there are alternatives, which orthomo-

Inositol and panthothenic acid
instead of sleeping pills

---

lecular physicians and nutritionally minded individuals are trying before resorting to drugs. Dr. Robert C. Atkins, author of *Dr. Atkins' Diet Revolution*, has his patients try pantothenic acid and about 2,000 mg. of inositol as sleep inducers instead of Seconal, Nembutal, Butisol, or other barbiturate sleeping pills. He has also had success using B_{15} to control blood sugar and B_{13} (oratic acid) to lower high blood pressure.

Before resorting to tranquilizers for your nerves, why not increase your ingestion of foods rich in B, and try a good stress B complex with C two to three times daily and see how you feel?

Garlic, vitamin C, and chicken soup have remarkable natural antibiotic and antihistamine properties.

Instead of becoming dependent upon commercial laxative preparations, why not try bran? (See sections 69 and 142.)

How about switching from commercial antacids to a multiple digestive enzyme? (See section 96.)

205. Vitamins Instead of Valium

Valium, a tranquilizer, is *the* most prescribed drug in the United States, according to *The New Handbook of Prescription Drugs*. Taken for a variety of conditions ranging from simple upsets and insomnia to angina pectoris, it is surely one of the most overused drugs around. (Based on weight it is also the most expensive drug on the U.S. market.)

Natural, nonaddictive tryptophan
can help you sleep.

If you're interested in breaking a Valium habit, in finding a nonaddictive natural substitute that will allow you to relax and to sleep, you and your doctor should look into L-tryptophan, an essential amino acid and constituent of all protein foods.

Research at Tufts University and the Sleep Laboratory of the Boston State Hospital has shown that L-tryptophan not only aids in building proteins, but is used by the brain to synthesize the vital brain chemical serotonin— a neuro-transmitter that carries messages between neurons, and one of the biochemical mechanisms of sleep. And that even a 1-g. dose (the tryptophan content of a large meal) can reduce the time it takes to fall asleep and increase time spent sleeping. Also, unlike sleeping medications, tryptophan does not alter the normal stages and cycles of sleep. A tryptophan supplement (2 g.) should be taken a half hour before bedtime with water or juice (no protein); a vitamin B_6 (50 mg.) and chelated magnesium (133 mg.)

Then, too, Adelle Davis called calcium and magnesium taken in a 2 to 1 ratio, "nature's tranquilizers." Many people who've tried them agree.

206. The Great Medicine Rip-off

More than ever before, Americans are gulping down drugs. What most people don't realize is that a lot of these medications—prescription as well as over-the-counter—are taking as much as they're giving, at least nutritionally. All too often the drugs either stop the absorption of nutrients or interfere with the cells' ability to use them.

A recent study showed that ingredients found in common over-the-counter cold, pain, and allergy remedies actually lowered the blood level of vitamin A. Since vitamin A protects and strengthens the mucous membranes lining the nose, throat, and lungs, a deficiency could give bacteria a cozy home to multiply in, prolonging the illness the drug was meant to alleviate.

> Aspirin can *triple* the excretion
> rate of vitamin C.

Aspirin, the household wonder drug, the most common ingredient in pain relievers, cold and sinus remedies, is a vitamin-C thief. Even a small amount can *triple* the excretion rate of vitamin C from the body. It can also lead to a deficiency of folic acid, which could cause anemia as well as digestive disturbances.

Corticosteroids (cortisone, prednisone), used for easing arthritis pain, skin problems, blood and eye disorders, and asthma, have been found to be related to lowered zinc levels. (See section 64.)

According to a study that appeared in the *Postgraduate Medical Journal,* a significant number of people who take barbiturates have low calcium levels.

Laxatives and antacids, taken by millions, have been found to disturb the body's calcium and phosphorus metabolism. And any laxative taken to excess can deplete large amounts of potassium.

Diuretics, commonly prescribed for high blood pressure, and antibiotics are also potassium thieves.

The following is a list of drugs that induce vitamin deficiencies and the vitamins they deplete. Look it over before you take your next medicine.

DRUGS THAT INDUCE VITAMIN DEFICIENCIES

Three basic mechanisms exist by which drugs induce vitamin deficiencies:

A. Impaired vitamin absorption
B. Impaired vitamin utilization
C. Enhanced vitamin elimination

A. IMPAIRMENT OF VITAMIN ABSORPTION

Drug	Vitamins depleted
Glutethimide (Doriden)	Folic acid
Cholestyramine (Cuemid, Questran)	A, D, E, K, and B_{12}
Os-Cal-Mone	B_6
Mineral oil	A, D, E, and K
Polysporin, Neo-Sporin, Neomycin, Mycolog, Neo-Cortef, Cortisporin, Lidosporin, Mycifradin	K, B_{12}, and folic acid
Kanamycin (Kantrex)	K and B_{12}
Tetracycline (Achromycin, Sumycin, Tetracyn)	K, calcium, magnesium, and iron

A. IMPAIRMENT OF VITAMIN ABSORPTION

Drug	Vitamins depleted
Chloramphenical (Chloromycetin)	K
Polymyxin (Aerosporin)	K
Sulfonamides	K
Phazyme	K
Sulfasalazine (Azulfidine, Aso-Gantanol, Gantanol)	Folic acid
Colchicine, Colbenemid	B_{12}, A, and potassium
Trifluoperazine (Stelazine)	B_{12}
Cortisone (tablets and suspension, Orasone, prednisone)	B_6, D, C, zinc, and potassium
Cathartic agents (Epsom Salts)	B_2, K
(Atromid-S) Clofibrinate	K
Antacids (Maalox, Mylanta, Gelusil, Tums, Rolaids, etc).	A and B

B. IMPAIRMENT OF VITAMIN UTILIZATION

Drug	Vitamins depleted
Coumarins (Dicumarol, Coumadin) y	K
Pro-Banthine, Probital	K
Methotrexate	Folic acid
Triamterene (Dyrenium)	Folic acid
Pyrimethamine (Daraprim)	Folic acid
Trimethoprim (Bactrim, Septra)	Folic acid
Nitrofurantoin (Furadantin, Macrodantin)	Folic acid
Phenylbutazone (Butazolidin)	Folic acid
Aspirin	Folic acid, C, and B_1
Indomethacin (Indocin)	B_1 and C
Bentyl with Phenobarb, Cantil with Phenobarb, Isordil with Phenobarb	K

C. ENHANCED VITAMIN EXCRETION

Drug	Vitamins depleted
Aldactazide, Aldactone	Potassium
Isoniazid (Inh, Nydrazid)	B_6

Drug	Vitamins depleted
Hydralazine (Apresoline)	B_6
Ser-Ap-Es (Serpasil, Apresoline, and Esidrix)	B_6
Penicillamine (Cuprimine)	B_6
Chlorothiazide (Diuril, Diupres)	Magnesium and potassium
Boric Acid	B_2
Bronkotabs, Bronkolixer	K
Chardonna	K

DRUGS WITH MULTIPLE MECHANISMS

Drug	Vitamins depleted
Diethylstilbestrol (DES)	B_6
Anticonvulsants	Folic acid and D
Phenytoin (Dilantin)	Folic acid and D
Barbiturates (Phenobarb, Seconal, Nembutal, Amytal, Butisol, Tuinal)	Folic acid and D
Oral contraceptive steroids (Brevicon, Demulen, Enovid, Lo-Ovral, Norinyl, Ovral)	Folic acid, C, and B_6
Alcohol	B_1, folic acid, and K
Betapar	B_6, C, zinc, and potassium

207. Marijuana and Cocaine

One joint can lower your
vitamin-C levels.

Over 45 million Americans have smoked marijuana. Medically, as well as socially, alcohol is more dangerous; but nutritionally marijuana is still right up there with the other vitamin raiders. Though the only substantial bodily changes that have been noted so far are a blood pressure rise, a temporary heartbeat increase, a lowering of body temperature, and, sometimes, a reddening of the eyes, the smoking of one joint can lower the vitamin-C level in your blood.

All smoking is bad for you, and marijuana smoking has the added disadvantage of getting you in trouble with the law in many states. But if you do smoke, be sure you're taking a vitamin-C supplement, 1,000 mg. A.M. and P.M. (time release) would be best, as well as vitamin E, 100 to 400 IU daily, to protect your lungs.

Cocaine, one of the most expensive drugs being used recreationally today, also has nutritional as well as legal drawbacks. Though not physically addictive, the drug, which stimulates the central nervous system, is metabolized rapidly, and the user is tempted to take another dose to maintain the high, creating strong drug dependence.

Cocaine speeds up the heart, increases the pulse, elevates blood pressure and body temperature, and prolonged use can damage the nasal tissues. If you can afford this dangerous habit, you'd be wise to invest in a good supply of supplements. Vitamin C, 1,000 mg. A.M. and P.M. (time release), is strongly recommended, along with a stress B complex, 50 mg. Because cocaine is an appetite depressant, you're probably skipping meals and losing nutrients that way also. A good multiple-vitamin and mineral tablet as well as a high-potency multiple mineral taken twice daily is also advised.

XXII

Losing It— Diets by the Pound

208. The Atkins Diet

This diet ignores calorie content and focuses on carbohydrate restriction; but unlike other low-carbohydrate programs, Dr. Atkins' calls for *no* carbohydrates (at least for the first week). By doing this, the body begins to throw off ketones (tiny carbon fragments that are by-products of incompletely burned fat) in amounts sufficient to account for substantial weight loss. According to Dr. Atkins, because carbohydrates are the first fuel your body burns for energy, if none are taken in then the body will draw upon stored fat for fuel. And as ketones are excreted, hunger as well as weight will disappear.

The pros and cons are many, but if you are

on this diet, Dr. Atkins recommends a high-potency vitamin supplement. I would suggest following the nsp program outlined in section 101, and taking an additional 1,000 mg. vitamin C with bioflavonoids if you've cut out all citrus fruit. Also at least 50 mg. B complex with morning and evening meal, 1 g. potassium divided over three meals, and 400 to 800 mcg. folic acid daily.

209. The Stillman Diet

Dr. Irwin Stillman's Quick Weight Loss Diet, often called "The Water Diet" because it requires drinking eight glasses of water daily, is essentially an all-protein program—no fats or carbohydrates. It permits no vegetables or fruits, no dairy products or grains, and is said to burn up about 275 more calories daily than a diet that contains the same number of calories but includes other elements, such as carbohydrates and fats. You don't count calories, but you're not supposed to stuff yourself either, and the average weight loss is said to be between five and fifteen pounds per week.

Even Dr. Stillman recognized the need for supplementation while on his diet. He recommended a multivitamin-mineral tablet for anyone following his regimen, and a high-potency multivitamin-mineral tablet for anyone on it who is over forty or eating very small amounts of food.

My own feeling is that anyone on Dr. Stillman's all-protein regimen should be taking a high-potency vitamin and chelated mineral tablet twice daily, along with 1,000 mg. vitamin C complex (time release) and a high-potency multiple chelated mineral tablet. Also, because the heavy water intake tends to flush the B vitamins as well as C from the body more quickly, a time-release vitamin B complex would be advisable, as would 400 to 800 mcg. folic acid and 1 g. potassium divided over three meals.

210. The Scarsdale Diet

This fourteen-day crash diet, on which you can lose up to twenty pounds, was created by Dr. Herman Tarnower and made famous in his book *The Complete Scarsdale Medical Diet* (Rawson, Wade Publishers, Inc.). It is basically a variation on the low-calorie, low-fat, low-carbohydrate, high-protein regimen. The difference between the Scarsdale diet and the Stillman and Atkins diets is that Dr. Tarnower has added a no-decision factor to his plan. In other words, you eat exactly what's on the menu for each meal every day. And no switching, at least not for two weeks.

Taking all responsibility from the dieter—except that of following instructions—has made the Scarsdale a popular and effective regimen.

As with any diet, because of the sudden cut in food intake, supplements are advised. A basic nsp (see section 101) should be taken if you're on the Scarsdale. Also recommended are vitamin E (dry form), 200 to 400 IU daily, and a good B complex.

274

211. Weight Watchers

This is a long-term regimen that advocates three meals a day with measured portions of protein, carbohydrates, and fat.

Though the program is nutritionally well rounded, most Weight Watchers that I've met agree that supplements have helped them keep up their energy levels while their calorie intake goes down. A multivitamin-mineral tablet, a multiple chelated mineral, and a vitamin C complex, 500 to 1,000 mg. taken one to two times daily should fill the bill.

212. The Drinking Man's Diet

This is another low-carbohydrate, high-fat and high-protein diet, but with the added appeal of allowing alcohol to be part of the regimen. Allegedly based on the Air Force diet (the Air Force denies), this one advocates keeping your carbohydrate count to 60 g. a day.

The diet states specifically that it is for healthy people, and cautions adherents to get at least 30 g. of carbohydrates daily and enough vitamin C.

Anyone on this diet would be well advised to take a vitamin-C supplement, along with a general nsp (see section 101) regimen, and B complex three times a day because of the alcohol.

213. Liquid Protein Diet

This diet is potentially dangerous. Substituting liquid protein for one or two meals is all right, but to do it for all three can be harmful. The liquid protein, which has no carbohydrates or fats, has been known to cause a potassium deficiency (among others), which can lead to severe illness—even death.

Your body needs nutrients to use nutrients, and liquid protein is *not* a total food. Even if you use it as a substitute for only two meals a day, be sure you're taking supplements. An nsp (see section 101) regimen, an extra 1,000 mg. vitamin C complex, and a 50 mg. B complex twice daily, and 1 g. potassium divided between the three meals would benefit the pound-droppers on this diet.

214. Zen Macrobiotic Diet

Contrary to popular belief, this diet is not connected with the Zen Buddhists, but is the creation of a Japanese man named George Ohsawa. Though it has gained many adherents, it is nutritionally dangerous when strictly followed.

There are ten stages to the diet, and milk is prohibited. You start by giving up dessert and work backwards until you're in the highest stage and eating nothing but grains, preferably brown rice. The diet, based on the oriental yin/yang philosophy, restricts fluid intake, which is dangerous, as is the lack of nutrients provided in meals consisting of nothing but brown rice. Followers believe that if your thoughts are right you can produce vitamins, minerals, and proteins within your own body, and actually change one element to another.

Just in case your thoughts aren't always

right, it would be advisable if you are on this diet, or just a strict vegetarian one, to take supplements. A high-potency vegetarian multiple-vitamin and mineral tablet twice daily along with a good B complex with folic acid is recommended. Also vitamin B_{12}, 100 mcg. one to three times a day.

215. Fructose Diet

This fourteen-day diet is for people who crave sweets. The secret is a supplement of fructose, a natural sugar, that not only satisfies your hunger and keeps up your energy, but allows you to lose a pound a day.

Developed by Dr. J.T. Cooper, the fructose diet is basically a low-calorie program, but by taking 36 to 42 g. of fructose a day you are supposed not to crave food. Unlike other dietary sugars, fructose doesn't require insulin to enter the body's cells. It is absorbed directly, eliminating the hypoglycemic (low blood sugar) reaction brought on by excess insulin, which is what makes dieters feel hungry.

Fructose is obtained from vegetables such as artichokes and corn. It is available in powder, flavored 2-g. chewable tablets, and syrup.

Ten glasses of water daily are recommended along with supplements. An nsp (see section 101) is important, as is potassium, 99 mg. (elemental) taken three times a day—one tablet with each meal.

216. Kelp, Lecithin, Vinegar, B_6 Diet

This low-profile but effective diet has been around for more than seven years and seems still to be popular. The basic components of the diet can be obtained in a tablet that contains kelp, lecithin, apple cider vinegar, and vitamin B_6. There are two potencies available: single and double strength. (With the single strength you take two tablets with each meal and with the double strength you take one.)

As with any diet that cuts down caloric intake, a good multiple-vitamin and mineral tablet taken with breakfast and dinner is recommended. Also a B complex and 1,000 mg. vitamin C (time release) twice daily.

217. Mindell Dieting Tips

• Before starting any diet, check with your physician. If you don't feel that your family doctor understands your dieting needs, contact a bariatrician, who specializes in the field. For the name of one in your area, write to the American Society of Bariatric Physicians, Suite 300, 5200 South Quebec, Englewood, Colorado 80111.

• If you're on a low- or no-carbohydrate diet, beware of artificially sweetened "sugarless" or "dietetic" gum or candy that has sorbitols, mannitols, or hexitols. These ingredients are metabolized in the system as carbohydrates, only more slowly.

• If you're on a diet that allows alcohol, a glass of wine before dinner stimulates the gastric juices and aids in proper digestion.

• Watch out for such diet fallacies as:

Gelatin dessert is nonfattening.
Grapefruit causes you to lose weight.

Fruits have no calories.
High-protein foods have no calories.
A pound of steak is not as fattening as a potato.
Toast has much fewer calories than bread.

• Whatever you're eating, sit down to eat it, and eat it slowly. (You might expend more calories standing than sitting, but you tend to eat more that way, too.)

• When selecting fruit, remember that all fruits are not equal, that an apple, a banana, or a pear has more calories and carbohydrates than a half cantaloupe, a cup of raw strawberries, or a fresh tangerine.

• When choosing your vegetable, take green beans instead of peas (you save 41 calories on a half-cup serving), spinach instead of mixed vegetables (you save 35 calories), and mashed potatoes—if you must—instead of hashed browns (you save 139 calories).

• Carbohydrate watchers, don't underestimate onions; one cup of cooked onions has 18 g.

• If you're counting every calorie, realize that 1 tablespoon of lecithin granules contains 50 calories and a lecithin capsule about 8.

• Try a one-day-a-week water fast (the ancient Greeks did it). Limit yourself to cold tap water (not iced) or herb tea with lemon or lime juice. Nothing else. This should pep you up, too.

218. Mindell Vitamin-balanced Diet to Lose and Live By

I know your mother told it to you, but it is true anyway—breakfast *is* the most important meal of the day. It comes after the longest period of time that you've been without food, and you cannot catch up nutritionally by eating a good lunch or dinner later.

If you're dieting, it is especially important to perk up your energy level at the start of the day. Even if you're in a hurry. And since most people I know are rushed in the morning, I advise the following blender breakfast:

BREAKFAST

8 oz. nonfat or low-fat milk (or juice)
A flavored low-calorie protein powder that contains nutritional yeast, lecithin, and fructose
4 ice cubes
Mix well in blender for 60 seconds. Calories, approximately: 150

This mixture can be frozen and used as a dessert for dinner or a pick-me-up snack if your calories quotient allows.

Lunch is a tricky meal. Fast-food restaurants are seductively convenient, and nothing blows a diet faster than "a few French fries" and a "tiny milkshake." If you really want to lose weight, think more along these lines:

LUNCH

Monday, Wednesday, Saturday, and Sunday

A modest portion (3–5 ounces) of water-packed canned or fresh fish, a large raw vegetable salad (with lemon or vinegar dressing), and a piece of fruit

2 eggs (prepared without fat) or cottage or pot cheese (no more than 1 cup), raw vegetables, 1 slice of bread with a light coating of margerine, and a fruit for dessert. (The American Heart Association suggests only 3 whole eggs per week, though many doctors allow more. Check with your own physician.)

Dinner is usually a dieter's downfall, but it doesn't have to be that way:

DINNER

Five nights a week you should have fish (sole, trout, salmon, halibut, etc.) or poultry broiled, boiled, or roasted (remove skin before eating poultry); and two nights a week you can have meat, once again broiled, boiled, or roasted; a cooked vegetable, a large salad (no more than 1 teaspoon oil in the dressing), a small boiled or baked potato once or twice a week, and a fresh fruit for dessert.

Stay away from alcohol—try sparkling mineral water with lime instead. As for other beverages, herb teas and plain old water are best.

Take your supplements six days a week and rest on the seventh. By doing this, you'll never have to worry about a build-up of fat-soluble vitamins in the system.

Time-release multiple vitamin with chelated minerals (at least 50 mg. B_1, B_2, and B_6, per tablet) taken A.M. and P.M.

Time-release vitamin C, 1,000 mg. with rose hips bioflavonoids, 2 tablets taken A.M. and P.M.

A multiple chelated mineral tablet with at least 500 mg. calcium and 250 mg. magnesium per tablet (must also have manganese, zinc, iron, selenium, chromium, copper, iodine, and potassium) taken A.M. and P.M.

Dry vitamin E, 400 IU—D-alpha-tocopherol with selenium, chromium, vitamin C, and ascorbates taken A.M. and P.M.

RNA 100 mg.—DNA 100 mg., 3 tablets daily, 6 days a week

Lecithin, 1,200 mg. (6 capsules) daily. (If you use lecithin granules in breakfast drink, this supplement is not necessary.)

Vitamin B_{15}, 50 mg. in the A.M.

XXIII

So You Think You Don't Eat Much Sugar and Salt

219. Kinds of Sugars

More than a hundred substances that qualify as sweet can be called sugars. The ones we come in contact with most often are *fructose*, a natural sugar found in fruit and honey; *glucose*, the body's blood sugar and the simplest form of sugar in which a carbohydrate is assimilated; *dextrose*, made from cornstarch and chemically identical to glucose; *lactose*, milk sugar; *maltose*, the sugar formed from the starch by the action of yeast; and *sucrose*, the sugar that is obtained from sugar cane or beets and refined to the product that reaches us as granules.

> Brown sugar is merely sugar crystals
> coated with molasses syrup.

Brown sugar, which many people assume to be healthier than white sugar, is merely sugar crystals coated with molasses syrup. (In the United States most brown sugar is made by simply spraying refined white sugar with the molasses syrup.) Raw sugar is banned in the United States because it contains contaminants. When it's partially refined and cleaned up, it can be sold as turbinado sugar. Honey is a blend of fructose and glucose. And then there are the various corn sweeteners, derived from cornstarch and composed mainly of dextrose, maltose, and the more complex sugars.

220. Dangers of Too Much Sugar

> Ketchup has 8 percent more sugar
> than ice cream.

The big problem with sugar is that we eat too much of it (over 128 pounds [30 teaspoons] per person in 1977) and often don't even know it. All carbohydrate sweeteners qualify as sugar, even though they may be called by other names; and when sucrose is the number-three ingredient on a box of cereal, corn syrup number five, and honey number seven, you don't realize it but you're eating something that is 50 percent sugar!

The consumer today is hooked on sugar right

from the start. Baby formulas are sweetened with sugar, as are many baby foods. Because sugar also acts as a preservative, retains and absorbs moisture, it's often in products we never think of as containing it, products such as salt, peanut butter, canned vegetables, bouillon cubes, and more. Would you believe that the ketchup you put on your hamburger has just less than 8 percent more sugar than ice cream? That cream substitute for coffee is 65 percent sugar compared to 51 percent for a chocolate bar? According to *Consumer Reports*, March 1978, there is 8.8 percent sugar in Coca-Cola and 13.7 percent in Dannon blueberry low-fat yogurt.

The fact is, we're eating too much sugar for our health. It is beyond argument that sugar is a prime factor in tooth decay. Also, one-third of our population is overweight, and obesity increases the possibility of heart disease, diabetes, hypertension, gallstones, back problems, and arthritis. Not that sugar alone is the cause, but its presence in foods induces you to eat more, and if you cut your calorie count without cutting your sugar intake, you'll lose nutrients faster than pounds. Sugar is also the villain where hypoglycemia is concerned, and, though there have been arguments pro and con, directly or indirectly a factor in diabetes and heart disease.

221. How Sweet It Is

Hidden sugars are where you least expect them, as the following table shows. If you want to be a sugar detective, my advice is to check labels. Look for sucrose substitutes such as corn syrup or corn sugar, and watch out for words ending in "-ose," which indicates the presence of sugar. A sugar by any name is still a sugar. And remember that not even medicines are immune from added sweeteners! (Ask your pharmacist if you want to be sure.)

SO YOU THINK YOU DON'T EAT MUCH SUGAR

Here are the approximate amounts of sugar, hidden in popular foods, either as an additive or naturally present.

FOOD ITEM	SIZE PORTION	APPROXIMATE EQUIVALENT IN TEASPOONFULS OF GRANULATED SUGAR
Beverages		
Cola drinks	1 (6-oz. bottle or glass)	3½
Cordials	1 (¾-oz. glass)	1½
Ginger ale	6 oz.	5
Highball	1 (6-oz. glass)	2½
Orangeade	1 (8-oz. glass)	5
Root beer	1 (10-oz. bottle)	4½
Seven-Up	1 (6-oz. bottle or glass)	3¾
Soda pop	1 (8-oz. bottle)	5
Sweet cider	1 cup	6
Whiskey sour	1 (3-oz. glass)	1½
Cakes and cookies		
Angel food	1 (4-oz. piece)	7
Applesauce cake	1 (4-oz. piece)	5½
Banana cake	1 (2-oz. piece)	2
Cheesecake	1 (4-oz. piece)	2

Food item	Size portion	Approximate equivalent in teaspoonfuls of granulated sugar
Cakes and cookies		
Chocolate cake (plain)	1 (4-oz. piece)	6
Chocolate cake (iced)	1 (4-oz. piece)	10
Coffee cake	1 (4-oz. piece)	4½
Cupcake (iced)	1	6
Fruit cake	1 (4-oz. piece)	5
Jelly roll	1 (2-oz. piece)	2½
Orange cake	1 (4-oz. piece)	4
Pound cake	1 (4-oz. piece)	5
Sponge cake	1 (1-oz. piece)	2
Brownies (unfrosted)	1 (¾ oz.)	3
Chocolate cookies	1	1¾
Fig Newtons	1	5
Gingersnaps	1	3
Macaroons	1	6
Nut cookies	1	1½
Oatmeal cookies	1	2
Sugar cookies	1	1½
Chocolate eclair	1	7
Cream puff	1	2
Doughnut (plain)	1	3
Doughnut (glazed)	1	6
Candies		
Average chocolate milk bar	1 (1½ oz.)	2½
Chewing gum	1 stick	½
Chocolate cream	1 piece	2
Butterscotch chew	1 piece	1
Chocolate mints	1 piece	2
Fudge	1-oz. square	4½
Gumdrop	1	2
Hard candy	4 oz.	20
Lifesavers	1	⅓
Peanut brittle	1 oz.	3½
Canned fruits and juices		
Canned apricots	4 halves and 1 tsp. syrup	3½

Food item	Size portion	Approximate equivalent in teaspoonfuls of granulated sugar
Canned fruits and juices		
Canned fruit juices (sweet)	½ cup	2
Canned peaches	2 halves and 1 tsp. syrup	3½
Fruit salad		
Fruit syrup	½ cup	3½
Fruit syrup	2 tsp.	2½
Stewed fruits	½ cup	2
Dairy products		
Ice cream	⅛ pt. (3½ oz.)	3½
Ice cream cone	1	3½
Ice cream soda	1	5
Ice cream sundae	1	7
Malted milk shake	1 (10-oz. glass)	5
Jams and jellies		
Apple butter	1 tsp.	1
Jelly	1 tsp.	4–6
Orange marmalade	1 tsp.	4–6
Peach butter	1 tsp.	1
Strawberry jam	1 tsp.	4
Desserts, miscellaneous		
Apple cobbler	½ cup	3
Blueberry cobbler	½ cup	3
Custard	½ cup	2
French pastry	1 (4-oz. piece)	5
Fruit gelatin	½ cup	4½
Apple pie	1 slice (average)	7
Apricot pie	1 slice	7
Berry pie	1 slice	10
Butterscotch pie	1 slice	4
Cherry pie	1 slice	10
Cream pie	1 slice	4
Lemon pie	1 slice	7
Mincemeat pie	1 slice	4
Peach pie	1 slice	7
Prune pie	1 slice	6

Food item	Size portion	Approximate equivalent in teaspoonfuls of granulated sugar
Desserts, miscellaneous		
Pumpkin pie	1 slice	5
Rhubarb pie	1 slice	4
Banana pudding	½ cup	2
Bread pudding	½ cup	1½
Chocolate pudding	½ cup	4
Cornstarch pudding	½ cup	2½
Date pudding	½ cup	7
Fig pudding	½ cup	7
Grapenut pudding	½ cup	2
Plum pudding	½ cup	4
Rice pudding	½ cup	5
Tapioca pudding	½ cup	3
Berry tart	1 cup	10
Blancmange	½ cup	5
Brown Betty	½ cup	3
Plain pastry	1 (4-oz. piece)	3
Sherbet	½ cup	9
Syrups, sugars, and icings		
Brown sugar	1 tsp.	3*
Chocolate icing	1 oz.	5
Chocolate sauce	1 tsp.	3½
Corn syrup	1 tsp.	3*
Granulated brown sugar	1 tsp.	3*
Honey	1 tsp.	3*
Karo syrup	1 tsp.	3*
Maple syrup	1 tsp.	5*
Molasses	1 tsp.	3½*
White icing	1 oz.	5*

*Actual sugar content.

222. A Balanced Program for Hypoglycemia*

BREAKFAST

(the most important meal of the day)

Any 2 proteins. Examples: natural cheese,
  eggs, fish, meat, poultry, cottage
  cheese
    Fresh fruits
    Herb teas or milk
    Whole-grain bread, optional, or
    Protein drink

RECIPE FOR HYPOGLYCEMIC'S PROTEIN DRINK

¼ tsp. kelp powder or granules
1 tsp. lecithin powder
½ tsp. niacin powder
1 tsp. vitamin-C powder
1 tsp. polyunsaturated vegetable oil (example: safflower)
1 tsp. nutritional yeast
1 tsp. bonemeal powder
1 tsp. acidophilus
1 tbs. glandular meat powder
½ tsp. cod liver oil
1 tsp. vitamin-E powder or 1 dry vitamin E 400 IU
2 balanced B-50 mg. tabs to put into drink
¼ tsp. inositol powder or 4 250 mg. tablets

*This program is not prescriptive. It is offered to the reader as a suggestion only. Check with a physician for hypoglycemia tests and symptoms.

Combine with milk, fruit or vegetable juice in a blender. Blend for 1 minute at high speed. Drink 2 oz. or 4 tsp. every two hours. The protein drink constitutes a complete meal.

Every two hours have either:

Two oz. protein drink and digestive aid if needed, plus 250 mg. pantothenic acid, or

Small portion of any type of protein and digestive aid, and

Small portion of any type low-carbohydrate vegetable, raw or steamed, and

Small portion of fruit once daily if well tolerated, or

Six to 12 1-g. chewable protein tablets, sweetened with fructose if protein drink or protein foods are not available

Supplements: See section 182.

Important: Drink at least 6 glasses of water daily, one-half hour before or after meals.

Avoid at all costs! White sugar, except fruit sugar, white flour, tobacco, alcohol, regular tea, coffee, or cola and other "soft" drinks (diet soft drinks included), processed foods, and fried foods.

223. Dangers of Too Much Salt

Taking things with a grain of salt is all well and good, but eating things with it might be a different story. The average intake of sodium chloride (table salt) is 6 to 18 g. daily, but an intake over 14 is considered excessive.

Too much salt can cause hypertension (high blood pressure), which increases the chances of heart disease. It causes abnormal fluid retention, which can result in dizziness and swelling of the legs. Also it may cause potassium to be lost in the urine. And in addition, too much salt can harm you nutritionally by interfering with the proper utilization of protein foods.

224. High-Salt Traps

Just because you stay away from pretzels and snack foods and don't pour on the table salt doesn't mean you're not getting more salt than you should. Salt traps are as hidden from view as sugar ones.

If you want to keep your salt intake down:

• Avoid the use of baking soda, monosodium glutamate (MSG, Accent), and baking powder in food preparation.

• Stay away from laxatives, most of which contain sodium.

• Do not drink or cook with water treated by a home water softener; it adds sodium to the water.

• Look for the words SALT, SODIUM, or the the chemical symbol *Na* when reading food labels.

• Don't eat cured meat such as ham, bacon, corned beef, or frankfurters, sausage, shellfish, any canned or frozen meat, poultry, or fish to which sodium has been added.

• When dining out, ask for an inside cut of meat, or chops or steaks without added salt.

225. How Salty Is It?

APPROXIMATE SODIUM CONTENT OF COMMON FOODS

Item	Amount	Salt (mg.)
Pickle, dill	1 large	1,928
Frozen turkey three-course dinner (Swanson)	1 (17 oz.)	1,735
Soy sauce	1 tbsp.	1,320
Pancakes (Hungry Jack Complete)	3 pancakes 4 in. each	1,150
Chicken noodle soup (Campbell's)	10 oz.	1,050
Tomato soup (Campbell's)	10 oz.	950
Green beans, canned (Del Monte)	1 cup	925
Cheese, pasteurized, processed American (Kraft)	2 oz.	890
Baked red kidney beans (B and M)	1 cup	810
Pizza, frozen (Celeste)	4 oz.	656
Danish cinnamon roles w/raisins (Pillsbury)	1 serving	630
Pudding, instant chocolate (Jell-O)	½ cup	486
Bologna (Oscar Mayer)	2 slices	450
Tuna, in oil (Del Monte)	3 oz.	430
Frankfurter, beef (Oscar Mayer)	1	425

PART FOUR

LOOKING YOUR BEST FROM THE INSIDE OUT

XXIV

Staying Beautiful—
Staying Handsome

226. Vitamins for Healthy Skin

What you look like on the outside depends a lot on what you do for yourself on the inside. And as far as your skin is concerned, vitamins and proper nutrition are essential.

To look your best, make sure you're getting 55 to 65 g. of protein a day. Drink eight glasses of water daily (herbal teas can count for a few of them), and keep your milk and yogurt consumption restricted to the nonfat variety. Keep away from chocolate, nuts, dried fruits, fried foods, cola drinks, coffee, alcohol, cigarettes, and excessive salt. Also, do not use sugar. Small amounts of honey or blackstrap molasses will sweeten just as well and you'll look better for it.

A good start toward healthy, glowing skin is a daily protein drink. It can be taken in place of any meal, but it makes an especially good breakfast.

PROTEIN DRINK

6 oz. raw nonfat milk
1 tbsp. nutritional yeast powder (lots of B vitamins)
3 tbsp. acidophilus (promotes friendly bacteria)
1 tbsp. granulated lecithin (breaks down bumps or cholesterol under the skin)
2 tbsp. protein powder
½–1 tbsp. blackstrap molasses or honey
Carob powder, bananas, strawberries, or any fresh fruit for flavoring
Mix in blender. (Add 3–4 ice cubes, if desired.)

SUPPLEMENTS

Multiple-vitamin and mineral complex—1 daily
Take after any meal. Important for skin tone and nerve health.

B complex, 100 mg. (time release)—1 daily
Take after any meal. B_2 (riboflavin) and B_6 (pyridoxine) reduce facial oiliness and blackhead formation.

Vitamin A (dry form), 25,000 IU—2 daily for 6 days a week
Take 1 after breakfast and 1 after dinner. Maintains soft, smooth, disease-free skin. Builds resistance to infections.

Rose hips vitamin C, 500 mg. with bioflavonoids—4 daily
Take 1 after each meal and at bedtime. Aids

in preventing the spread of acne. Promotes healing of wounds, bruising, and scar tissue. Helps to prevent breakage of capillaries on face.

Vitamin E, 400 IU (dry form)—3 daily

Take 1 after each meal. Improves circulation in tiny face capillaries. Aids in healing by replacing cells on the skin's outer layer. Works with vitamin C in making skin less susceptible to acne. Use vitamin-E oil externally on skin for healing burns, abrasions, and scar tissue.

Multiple chelated minerals—6 daily

Take 2 tablets after each meal (or 3 in A.M. and P.M.). Helps maintain the acid–alkaline balance of the blood necessary for a clear complexion. Calcium is for soft, smooth skin tissue; copper for skin color; iron to improve pale skin; potassium for dry skin and acne; zinc for external and internal wound healing.

Choline and inositol, 1,000 mg.—4 tablets daily.

Take 2 after breakfast and dinner. (Lecithin granules, 2 tbsp. daily, can be substituted for choline and inositol tabs.) Helps emulsify cholesterol (fatty deposits or bumps under the skin). Purifies the kidneys which aids the skin.

Acidophilus—6 tbsp. daily

Take 2 tbsp. or 6 capsules after each meal. Helps fight skin eruptions caused by unfriendly bacteria in the system.

Chlorophyll—3 tsp. or 9 tablets daily

Take 1 tsp. or 3 tablets after each meal. Reduces hazard of bacterial contamination. Possesses antibiotic action. An excellent aid to wound healing, after washing thoroughly with a soap substitute made from the comfrey plant.

If the face is badly blemished, extra zinc is advised. Take six tablets daily, two after each meal. Aids in growth and repair of injured tissues.

227. Vitamins for Healthy Hair

Shampoos and conditioners are not enough. To make sure that you're giving your crowning glory its due, you have to be aware that nutrition plays a very important role in having terrific, shiny hair. Unlike the skin, hair cannot repair itself; but you *can* get new, healthier hair to grow.

The first thing to do is examine your diet. Does it include fish, wheat germ, yeast, and liver? It should. The vitamins and minerals that these foods supply are what your hair needs, along with frequent scalp massage, a good pH-balanced, protein-enriched shampoo, and supplements.

SUPPLEMENTS

Multiple-vitamin and mineral complex—1 daily
Take after any meal. Important for general health of hair.

B complex, 100 mg. (time release)—1 daily
Take after any meal. B vitamins are essential for hair growth. Adelle Davis found that pantothenic acid, folic acid, and PABA helped restore gray hair to its natural color.

Vitamin A, 25,000 IU—1–2 daily 6 days a week
Take A.M. and P.M. Works with vitamin B
to keep hair shiny.

Multiple chelated minerals—1 daily
Take with breakfast. Minerals such as silicon,
sulfur, iodine, and iron help prevent falling
hair.

Keep in mind that you need some fatty acids,
vitamin E, and choline in your body for vitamin
A to survive.

228. Vitamins for Hands and Feet

Your hands take lots of abuse. Detergents strip
away natural oils, and water and weather alone
can cause chapping. Rubber gloves are a good
idea, but if you already have splits in your skin
or some sort of dermatitis, they could *not* be
put directly on your hands. (A pair of cotton
gloves beneath the rubber ones will absorb
perspiration and prevent reinfection.) Also, do
not use cornstarch in the gloves; it can promote
the growth of micro-organisms. If you want to
use something to absorb the moisture, try
plain unscented talcum powder.

As for toenails and fingernails, the best remedy for problems is diet. Gelatin is commonly
accepted as the cure for weak nails, but this is
a misconception. The nails do need protein, but
gelatin is a poor supplier. Not only are two
essential amino acids missing, but another
amino acid, glycine, is supplied in amounts you
do not need. Foods rich in sulfur, such as egg
yolks, should be part of your diet, and desic-

cated liver (powder or tablets) should be taken
as a supplement.

SUPPLEMENTS

Multiple-vitamin and mineral complex—1 daily
   Take after any meal. Promotes general skin
   health and growth of nails.
B complex, 100 mg. (time release)—1 daily
   Take after any meal. Helps build resistance
   to fungus infections and vital to nail growth.
Vitamin A, 25,000 IU—1 daily 6 days a week
   Take after any meal. Helps to prevent split-
   ting nails.
Vitamin E, 100–400 IU—1–2 daily
   Take in A.M. and P.M. Necessary for proper
   utilization of vitamin A.
Multiple chelated minerals—1 daily
   Take after any meal. Iron helps strengthen
   brittle nails, zinc gets rid of white spots.

229. Natural Cosmetics—What's in Them

Many cosmetics nowadays are advertised as
"natural," but looking at the ingredients can
cause you to wonder. To be sure of what you're
getting, read the label carefully. The following
explanations of cosmetic ingredients should
make things clearer.

Amyl Dimethyl PABA—a sunscreening agent
   from PABA, a B-complex factor.
Annatto—a vegetable color obtained from the
   seeds of a tropical plant.
Avocado oil—a vegetable oil obtained from
   avocados

302

Caprylic/Capric triglyceride—an emollient obtained from coconut oil

Carrageenan—a natural thickening agent from dried Irish moss

Castor oil—an emollient oil collected from the pressing of castor bean seeds

Cetyl alcohol—a component of vegetable oils

Cetyl palmitate—a component of palm and coconut oils

Citric acid—a natural organic acid found widely in citrus plants

Cocamide DEA—a thickener obtained from coconut oil

Coconut oil—obtained by pressing the kernels of the seeds of the coconut palm

Decyl oleate—obtained from tallow or coconut oil

Disodium monolaneth-5-sulfosuccinate—obtained from lanolin and used to improve the texture of hair

Fragrance—oils obtained from flowers, grasses, roots, and stems that give off a pleasant or agreeable odor

Goat milk whey—protein-rich whey obtained from goat's milk

Glyceryl stearate—an organic emulsifier obtained from glycerin

Hydrogenated castor oil—a waxy material obtained from castor oil

Imidzaolidinyl urea—a preservative derived naturally as a product of protein metabolism (hydrolysis)

Lanolin alcohol—a constituent of lanolin that performs as an emollient and emulsifier

Laureth-3—an organic material obtained from coconut and palm oils

Methyl glucoside sesquistearate—an organic emulsifier obtained from a natural simple sugar

Mineral oil—an organic emollient and lubricant

Olive oil—a natural oil obtained from olives

Peanut oil—a vegetable oil obtained from peanuts

Pectin—derived from citrus fruits and apple peel

PEG lanolin—an emollient and emulsifier obtained from lanolin

Petrolatum—petroleum jelly

P.O.E. (20) methyl glucoside sesquistearate—an organic emulsifier from a simple natural sugar

Potassium sorbate—obtained from sorbic acid found in the berries of mountain ash

Safflower oil-hybrid—a natural emollient obtained from a strain of specially cultivated plants

Sesame oil—oil of pressed sesame seeds

Sodium cetyl sulfate—a detergent and emulsifier obtained from coconut oil

Sodium laureth sulfate—a detergent obtained from coconut oil

Sodium lauryl sulfate—a detergent obtained from coconut oil

Sodium PCA—a natural-occurring humectant found in the skin where it acts as the natural moisturizer

Sorbic acid—a natural preservative derived from berries of mountain ash

Tocopherol—a natural vitamin E

Undecylenamide DEA—a natural preservative derived from castor oil

230. Not So Pretty Drugs

Medications are necessary for certain conditions, but doctors often fail to mention their possible side effects. It is a rare physician who puts his patient on the pill and tells her that her face might break out, or that she might suffer hair loss; but many women on oral contraceptives find this out soon enough. In fact, many drugs can be the cause of skin and other cosmetic problems. The following is a list of just a few:

Amytal	Skin rash, swollen eyelids, itchy skin
Butisol	Acne, pimples
Dalmane	Rash, flushes
Dexamyl	Swollen patches, itchy skin
Dexedrine	Swollen patches, itchy skin
Equanil	Rash, welts, dermatitis
Librium	Pimples
Miltown	Welts, flaking skin, itching
Nembutal	Skin rash
Phenobarbital	Rash, itchy skin, swollen eyelids
Placidyl	Itchy skin, swollen patches
Quaalude	Pimples, welts
Talwin	Rash, facial swelling, skin peeling
Tetracycline	Taken during pregnancy and in infancy may cause permanent discoloration of child's teeth

Thorazine	Peeling skin, jaundice, welts, swelling
Tofranil	Rash, itchy skin, jaundice
Tuinal	Can aggravate existing skin condition
Valium	Jaundice, rash, swollen patches

XXV

Staying Young, Energetic, and Sexy

231. Retarding the Aging Process Through the Remarkable Nucleic Acids

Aging is caused by the degeneration of cells. Our bodies are made up of millions of these cells, each with a life of somewhere around two years or less. But before a cell dies, it reproduces itself. Why, then, you might wonder, shouldn't we look the same now as we did ten years ago? The reason for this is that with each successive reproduction, the cell goes through some alteration—basically, deterioration. So as our cells change, deteriorate, we grow old.

> You can look and feel six
> to twelve years younger.

Dr. Benjamin S. Frank, author of *Nucleic Acid Therapy in Aging and Degenerative Disease* (New York: Psychological Library, 1969; revised 1974), has found that deteriorating cells can be rejuvenated if provided with substances that directly nourish them—substances such as nucleic acids.

DNA (deoxyribonucleic acid) and RNA (ribonucleic acid) are our nucleic acids. DNA is essentially a chemical boiler-plate for new cells. It sends out RNA molecules like a team of well-trained workers to form them. When DNA stops giving the orders to RNA, new cell construction ceases—as does life. But by helping the body stay well supplied with nucleic acids, Dr. Frank has found that you can look and feel six to twelve years younger than you actually are.

According to Dr. Frank, we need 1 to 1½ g. of nucleic acid daily. Though the body can produce its own nucleic acids, he feels they are broken down too quickly into less useful compounds and should be supplied from external sources if the aging process is to be retarded, even reversed.

Foods rich in nucleic acids are wheat germ, bran, spinach, asparagus, mushrooms, fish (especially sardines, salmon, and anchovies), chicken liver, oatmeal, and onions. He recommends a diet where seafood is eaten seven times a week, along with two glasses of skimmed milk, a glass of fruit or vegetable juice, and four glasses of water daily.

After only two months of RNA-DNA supplementation and diet, Dr. Frank found that his patients had more energy and that there was a substantial diminution of lines and wrinkles, with healthier, rosier, and younger-looking skin in evidence.

232. Basic Vitamin-Mineral RNA-DNA Program

Along with proper diet, a good supplement regimen is important to the success of an RNA-DNA program. I've found that the following works best:

High-potency multiple vitamin with chelated minerals (time release preferred) A.M. and P.M.

Vitamin C, 1,000 mg. with bioflavonoids A.M. and P.M.

Vitamin E, 400 IU (dry form) with antioxidants A.M. and P.M.

RNA-DNA, 100-mg. tablets, 1 daily for one month, then 2 daily for the next month, then 3 daily thereafter, 6 days a week

Stress B complex A.M. and P.M.

233. High-Pep Energy Regimen

Whether you want to feel good, or just look good, exercise, diet, and the right supplements are the tickets to high energy.

If you're not into jogging, can't afford the

sneakers, don't play tennis, find yourself reluctant to swim in twenty-below weather, and hate calisthenics, I have the perfect exercise for you—jumping rope.

A jump rope is inexpensive, convenient (you can take it everywhere), and lots of fun to use. And it works! In terms of calories burned, jumping rope can outdo bicycling, tennis, and swimming. An average person of about 150 pounds uses up 720 calories an hour jumping rope (120 to 140 turns per minute). When you realize that an hour of tennis uses up only 420 calories, you have a better idea of just how good jumping rope can be for you.

For keeping energy high, remember to eat a combination of two protein foods (or a protein drink), at each meal; drink at least six glasses of water daily (a half hour before or after meals); avoid refined sugar, flour, tobacco, alcohol, tea, coffee, soft drinks, processed and fried foods.

A good pep-up protein drink:

2 tbsp. protein powder
1 tbsp. lecithin powder
2 tbsp. acidophilus liquid
1 tbsp. nutritional yeast
1 tbsp. safflower oil (optional)

Blend with milk, water, or juice in blender for 1 minute.

234. High-Pep Supplements

With breakfast:

High-potency multiple vitamin with chelated minerals (time release preferred)

310

2 stress B complex with C
Vitamin E, 400 IU
High-potency multiple chelated mineral
Acidophilus, 3 capsules or 2 tbsp. liquid
Lecithin powder, 1 tbsp. or 3 19-g. capsules
3 calcium and magnesium tablets

With lunch:

2 stress B complex with C
Vitamin E, 400 IU
Acidophilus, 3 capsules of 2 tbsp. liquid
Lecithin powder, 1 tbsp. or 3 19-g. capsules
Optional: vitamin B_{12}, liver tablets, digestive
   enzymes

With dinner:

2 stress B complex with C
Vitamin E, 400 IU
Acidophilus, 3 capsules or 2 tbsp. liquid
Lecithin powder, 1 tbsp. or 3 19-g. capsules
Optional: digestive enzymes

235. Vitamins and Sex

The important thing to remember is that if
you're not feeling up to par your sex drive is
going to suffer along with the rest of you.

There have been many claims for vitamin E
in relationship to sex. Studies have indeed
shown that it increases the fertility in males
and females and helps restore male potency.
That it strongly influences the sex drive in men
and women has yet to be proven, though I
have met many vitamin-E takers who are happily convinced that it does.

> The largest percentage of zinc
> in a man's body is found in
> the prostate.

Another noteworthy sex nutrient is zinc. The largest percentage of zinc in a man's body is found in the prostate, and a lack of the mineral can produce testicular atrophy and prostate trouble. (See section 64.)

Remember, vitamins that keep up your energy levels (see sections 233, 234) will also do a lot for your sexual performance.

236. Food and Supplements for Better Sex

Oysters (yes, they're high in zinc), shellfish of all kinds, brewer's yeast, wheat bran, wheat germ, whole grains, and pumpkin seeds. Incorporating these foods in a program that includes a high-protein and basically low-carbohydrate diet, exercise, and supplements is as good as an aphrodisiac for lovers.

SUPPLEMENTS

nsp (see section 101)
Vitamin B complex, 50 mg., 1–3 times daily
Vitamin E, 400 IU, 1–3 times daily
Zinc, 50 mg. (chelated), 1–3 times daily

XXVI
Traveling Healthy

237. Vitamins On the Go

Don't forget to pack the vitamins! Believe it or not, vitamins on vacation—or whatever your reason for traveling—are as important as they are at home. In many cases even more so. The stresses of travel, though they often go unnoticed, can be significant.

If you're traveling to warm or tropical places, be sure that the vitamins you take are in opaque containers and that you keep them in a cool place, not out in the sun. Pack a good sunscreening cream with PABA or a vitamin-E preparation (20,000 IU). If you have been taking vitamin-D supplements and want to get off for a while, this is the time. A wise choice of vitamins to bring along would be:

High-potency multiple vitamin and minerals
(take 1 with breakfast and dinner)
Vitamin E, 400 IU (dry form)
(take 1–2 daily)
Vitamin C, 1,000 mg. with bioflavonoids
(take with breakfast and dinner)
Stress B complex, 50 mg.
(take 2–3 times daily)

If you're headed to chillier environs, be sure to take plenty of vitamin C (time release recommended), and if you plan to be indoors a lot, vitamin D also. The vitamins listed above will work in any climate, but if you do find yourself in an area colder than you're used to, remember to take the vitamin C with all your meals instead of just breakfast and dinner.

> Acidophilus can be a traveler's
> best friend.

If you're traveling to foreign ports, keep in mind that acidophilus (3 capsules or 2 tablespoons liquid) three times a day is good for diarrhea prevention.

238. Are Foreign Vitamins Different?

Vitamins the world over are the same, only dosages vary. Read the label. The metric system is used internationally for measurement, and nutrients are measured by weight. (See section 80 for a better understanding of what equals what.) In the metric system, the energy value of food is measured in units called *joules*, or kilocalories, better known as calories. Four of our calories are the equivalent of 17 joules. In other words, a joule is slightly more than four times a calorie.

PART FIVE

VITAMINS FOR PETS

XXVII

Man's Best Friend
Deserves the Best

239. Vitamins for Your Dog

Dogs need vitamins as much as people do. Their requirements, of course, are not the same as ours, but they too need all the nutrients. (If you want to know exactly what they need for basic nutrition, write for the National Research Council's *Nutrient Requirements of Dogs*, National Academy of Sciences, Washington, D.C.)

An adult dog needs 4.4 g. protein daily, along with 1.3 g. fat, 0.4 g. linoleic or arachidonic acid, and 15.4 g. carbohydrate. Puppies need twice that amount.

Proteins are essential for a dog's growth and body repair. Those with a high biological value, such as eggs, muscle meat, fish meat, soybeans, milk, and yeast, are the best. If you want to give your dog eggs, be sure that they're cooked. Raw egg white contains avidin, which prevents biotin from being absorbed. Milk, though good for dogs, often causes diarrhea, so yogurt and cottage cheese are recommended.

Carbohydrates are used by dogs for energy, but it is suggested that no more than 50 to 60 percent of their food include them.

Fats, the most concentrated energy source, supply the essential fatty acid for healthy skin and hair. A deficiency can retard puppies' growth and lead to coarse hair and flaking skin. One teaspoon of safflower or corn oil added to the dog's dry food can help.

Imbalanced supplements can
harm your dog.

Calcium and phosphorus, in a ratio of 1.2 to 1, should be included in the dog's diet. If the ratio is incorrect, abnormal mineralization can occur in the bones of growing puppies as well as adult dogs. There must also be sufficient vitamin D for proper absorption of these two minerals. Because the balance is so important, *be certain that the vitamin supplements you give are balanced.* Too much bonemeal or cod liver oil can result in problems as severe as those you're trying to combat.

Cod liver oil is not advised as a routine supplement; it can lead to vitamin-D overload.

All-meat diets are not good for your pet because the calcium-phosphorus ratio is wrong and there are inadequate amounts of vitamins A, D, and E.

Brewer's yeast, mixed in with your dog's food, will help prevent fleas. (It works for cats too.) Fleas despise the odor it gives off after your dog ingests it.

Do not give your dog supplemental vitamins A, D, or niacin. They have an adverse effect on the animal. (See section 98 for "Cautions.")

240. Arthritis and Dysplasia Regimen for Dogs

Dogs, unlike humans, manufacture their own vitamin C, but recent research has shown that supplemental C can be effective in the treatment of arthritis and dysplasia. I recommend, though, that you consult your vet before starting any vitamin program. Ask him or her about this regimen:

Vitamin C, 300 mg.
4–5 alfalfa tablets
Vitamin E, 100 IU
Mix with food daily.

XXVIII
Keeping Kitty Fit

241. Vitamins for Your Cat

Cats need vitamins, just as people and dogs do, but nutritional requirements for them have not been as well established. (For the most recent available information, you can write for the National Research Council's *Nutrient Requirements of Laboratory Animals*, National Academy of Sciences, Washington, D.C.)

> Cow's milk is insufficient
> for a growing kitten.

Protein requirements for cats are high, considerably higher than those of dogs or people. And kittens need one-third more protein than adult cats. Muscle meats, organ meat, poultry, fish, cheese, eggs, and milk are all good sources. (Eggs should be cooked or, if given raw, only the yolk should be used.) If you are giving a kitten milk, use a dry powdered milk at double the concentation given a human baby; cow's milk isn't nutritious enough for an infant cat.

Carbohydrates are not actually required in a cat's diet, but they are used as energy. If there are adequate levels of fats and protein, 33 percent of the diet can be made up of carbohydrates.

Give your cat the fats
you shouldn't eat.

Fats are a cat's most concentrated source of energy. Unlike people, cats can have diets of up to 64 percent fat and show no signs of vascular problems. Only because fats are more costly than carbohydrates do most cat foods have low percentages. In fact, you can give your cat the fats you need to cut down on— butter, animal fat, vegetable. Where cats are concerned, polyunsaturates are not the good guys. Too much polyunsaturated fatty acid is antagonistic to vitamin E, and fat deposits in the cat's body can be seriously affected.

Although levels of all the essential vitamins haven't been established for cats, the importance of certain vitamins in a cat's diet should be noted. For example, cats are dependent on their diet for fully formed vitamin A. (Their requirement is much higher than that of dogs because unlike dogs they cannot manufacture vitamin A in the body from carotene.) On the other hand, too much vitamin A can result in bone deformities. Liver as a supplement (not a total diet) is recommended, as is a *balanced* vitamin-mineral preparation. Fish, butter, milk, and cheese are also high in vitamin A.

The B vitamins are also important for a cat's nerve stability, outer coat, and inner tissues. B_6 (pyridoxine) helps prevent urinary calculi, a serious problem for altered male cats. (A diet low in ash is recommended.) In general, cats require twice the amount of B vitamins needed by dogs, and feeding dog food to a cat for an extended period of time can result in a B-complex deficiency. It should also be noted that B_1 (thiamine) can be destroyed by an antagonist in raw fish. (For foods high in B vitamins, see sections 25, 26, 27, and 28.)

All-fish diets are not
healthy for cats.

Vitamin-E deficiency can occur from feeding excessive amounts of red meat tuna. (It can also occur because of any all-fish diet.) Lack of appetite, fever, pain, and a reluctance to move are characteristic symptoms of pansteatitis, which results from vitamin-E deficiency. If this occurs, see your vet, don't feed tuna unless it is supplemented with vitamin E, and don't use fish oils as supplements.

The calcium-phosphorus ratio in a cat's diet should be about one to one, with adequate amounts of vitamin D. Since manufacturers of canned cat foods usually add irradiated yeast, a source of vitamin D, supplements of D are unnecessary—and can be dangerous. (See section 98 for "cautions.")

A multiple vitamin with iron—prepared especially for cats—is often given for feline anemia. The disease is rare in cats on a balanced diet that includes cooked and raw muscle meat, organ meats, cooked or canned chicken and fish, vitamin-rich cereals, and vegetables.

Keep in mind that pregnant or lactating cats, who often eat 10 to 15 ounces of food a day, have double or triple the vitamin requirements of an average five-to seven-pound cat.

Afterword

As more and more people have become aware of the importance of vitamins in their daily lives, the need for clear, uncomplicated information has become evident. And with recent research showing that the right vitamins at the right time are much more important to us than anyone ever realized, the need has become a necessity. It is my hope that this book has fulfilled that need, that it has debunked the myths surrounding food and nutrition, and erased any uncertainties about the nature, function, and safety of vitamins.

Whether you have read the book cover to cover or simply thumbed through to personally relevant points, I believe you'll find its reference value will increase as new life situations arise. My intention was to provide an omnibus guide that could answer not only your present vitamin questions, but future ones as well. As time goes by, the sections on staying young, energetic and sexy and retarding the aging process will bear rereading, as will those offering regimens for whatever your new particular circumstance happens to be. In other words, the information I have set down is meant to be perused, and is intended not just for today, but for many, many happy and healthy tomorrows.

EARL L. MINDELL, *Pharm.B. R.Ph*

Los Angeles, Calif.
June 11, 1979

APPENDIX

BIBLIOGRAPHY AND RECOMMENDED READING

I owe a great debt of thanks to the many scientists, doctors, nutritionists, professors, and researchers whose painstaking and all too often unrewarding work in the field of vitamins and nutrition has made this book possible.

The following is given to show my sincere appreciation and make known the foundation upon which I have built my knowledge. Many of the books are highly technical and confusing for the layman, meant as they are for professionals in the field. But others, which I have marked with an asterisk, I heartily commend to you for further reading and a healthier future.

*Abrahamson, E.M., and Pezet, A.W. *Body, Mind and Sugar*. New York: Holt, Rinehart and Winston, 1951.

*Adams, Ruth. *The Complete Home Guide to All the Vitamins*. New York: Larchmont Books, 1972.

*Adams, Ruth, and Murray, Frank. *Minerals: Kill or Cure*. New York: Larchmont Books, 1976.

*Aguilar, Nona. *Totally Natural Beauty*. New York: Rawson Associates Publishers, 1977.

*Airola, Paavo. *Are You Confused?* Phoenix, AZ: Health Plus, 1972.

*———. *How to Get Well*. Phoenix, AZ: Health Plus, 1975.

*———. *Hypoglycemia, A Better Approach*. Phoenix, AZ: Health Plus, 1977.

Amberson, Rosanne. *Raising Your Cat*. New York: Bonanza Books, 1969.

*Atkins, Robert C. *Dr. Atkins' Diet Revolution*. New York: David McKay, 1972.

*Bailey, Hubert. *Vitamin E: Your Key to a Healthy Heart*. New York: ARC Books, 1964, 1966.

Bieri, John G. "Fat-soluble vitamins in the eighth revision of the Recommended Dietary Allowances." *Journal of the American Dietetic Association* 64 (February 1974).

Blood: The River of Life. American National Red Cross, 1976.

*Borsaak, Henry. *Vitamins: What They Are and How They Can Benefit You*. New York: Pyramid Books, 1971.

"Bread: You Can't Judge a Loaf by Its Color." *Consumer Reports* 41 (May 1976).

*Bricklin, Mark. *Practical Encyclopedia of Natural Healing*. Emmaus, PA: Rodale Press, 1976.

Brody, Jane E. "Cancer-blocking Agents Found in Foods." *The New York Times*, 6 March 1979.

*Burack, Richard, with Fox, Fred J. *New Handbook of Prescription Drugs*. New York: Pantheon Books, 1967.

Burton, Benjamin. *Human Nutrition*. 3rd ed. New York: McGraw-Hill, 1976.

"Buying Beef." *Consumer Reports* 39 (September 1974).

*Carr, William H.A. *The Basic Book of the Cat*. New York: Gramercy Publishing Co., 1963.

*Chapman, Esther. *How to Use the 12 Tissue Salts*. New York: Pyramid Books, 1977.

*Clark, Linda, *The Best of Linda Clark*. New Canaan, CT: Keats Publishing Co., 1976.

*———. *Know Your Nutrition*. New Canaan, CT: Keats Publishing Co., 1973.

*———. *Secrets of Health and Beauty*. New York: Jove Publications, 1977.

*Consumer Reports, Editors of. *The Medicine Show*. Mount Vernon, NY: Consumers Union, 1961.

Cooper, Barber, Mitchell, Rynberge, Green. *Nutrition in Health and Disease*. New York: Lippincott, 1963.

Cumulative Index for Journal of Applied Nutrition. La Habra, CA: International College of Applied Nutrition, 1947–76, 1976.

*Davis, Adelle. *Let's Eat Right to Keep Fit*. New York: Harcourt, Brace and World, 1954.

*———. *Let's Get Well*. New York: Harcourt, Brace and World, 1965.

*———. *Let's Have Healthy Children*. 2nd ed. New York: Harcourt, Brace and World, 1959.

*Dufty, William, *Sugar Blues*. Pennsylvania: Chilton Book Co., 1975.

*Ebon, Martin. *Which Vitamins Do You Need?* New York: Bantam Books, 1974.

Flynn, Margaret A. "The Cholesterol Controversy." *Journal of the American Pharmacy* NS18 (May 1978).

"Food Facts Talk Back." *Journal of the American Dietetic Association*, 1977.

*Frank, Benjamin S. *No-Aging Diet*. New York: Dial, 1976.

*Fredericks, Carlton. *Eating Right for You*. New York: Grosset and Dunlap, 1972.

*———. *Look Younger/Feel Healthier*. New York: Grosset and Dunlap, 1977.

*———. *Psycho Nutrients*. New York: Grosset and Dunlap, 1976.

*Gomez, Joan, and Gerch, Marvin J. *Dictionary of Symptoms*. New York: Stein and Day, 1968.

Goodhart, Robert S., and Shills, Maurice E. *Modern*

333

Nutrition in Health and Disease. 5th ed. Philadelphia: Lea and Febiger, 1973.

*Graedon, Joe. *The People's Pharmacy*. New York: St. Martin's Press, 1976.

Guidelines for the Eradication of Iron Deficiency Anemia. New York: International Nutritional Anemia Consultative Group (INACG) 1976.

Guidelines for the Eradication of Vitamin-A Deficiency and Xerophthalmia. International Vitamin-A Consultative Group (IVACG).

Harper, Alfred E. "Recommended Dietary Allowances: Are They What We Think They Are?" *Journal of the American Dietetic Association* 64 (February 1974).

Holvey, David, ed. *The Merck Manual*. 12th ed. Rahway, N.J.: Merck and Co., 1972.

Howe, Phyllis S. *Basic Nutrition in Health and Disease*. 6th ed. Philadelphia: W.B. Saunders Co., 1976.

"How Nutritious Are Fast-Food Meals?" *Consumer Reports* (May 1975).

*Hunter, B.T. *The Natural Foods Primer*. New York: Simon and Schuster, 1972.

Index of Nutrition Education Materials. Washington, D.C.: Nutrition Foundation, 1977.

Journal of Applied Nutrition. International College of Applied Nutrition, La Habra, CA, 1974–76.

*Karelitz, Samuel. *When Your Child Is Ill*. New York: Random House, 1969.

Katz, Marcella. *Vitamins, Food, and Your Health*. Public Affairs Committee, 1971, 1975.

*Kordel, L. *Health Through Nutrition*. New York: MacFadden-Bartell, 1971.

*Linde, Shirley. *The Whole Health Catalog*. New York: Rawson Associates Publishers, 1977.

*Lucas, Richard. *Nature's Medicines*. New York: Prentice-Hall, 1966.

*McGinnis, Terri. *The Well Cat Book*. New York: Random House-Bookworks, 1975.

*——. *The Well Dog Book*. New York: Random House-Bookworks, 1974.

"Marijuana: The Health Questions." *Consumer Reports* 40 (March 1975).

*Martin, Clement G. *Low Blood Sugar: The Hidden*

Menace of Hypoglycemia. New York: Arco Publishing Co., 1976.

Martin, Marvin. Great Vitamin Mystery. Rosemont, IL: National Dairy Council, 1978.

*Mayer, Jean. A Diet for Living. New York: David McKay, 1975.

Mitchell, Helen S. "Recommended Dietary Allowances Up to Date." Journal of the American Dietetic Association 64 (February 1974).

National Health Federation Bulletin. November 1978.

National Research Council. Recommended Dietary Allowances. 8th ed., revised. Washington, DC: National Academy of Sciences, 1974.

National Research Council. Toxicants Occurring Naturally in Foods. 2nd ed. Washington, DC: National Academy of Sciences, 1973.

*Newbold, H.L. Dr. Newbold's Revolutionary New Discovery About Weight Loss. New York: Rawson Associates Publishers, 1977.

*———. Mega-Nutrients for Your Nerves. New York: Peter H. Wyden, Publisher, 1978.

*Null, Gary. The Natural Organic Beauty Book. New York: Dell, 1972.

*Null, Gary and Steve. The Complete Book of Nutrition. New York: Dell, 1972.

*Nutrition Almanac. New York: McGraw-Hill, 1973.

Nutrition—Applied Personally. La Habra, CA: International College of Applied Nutrition, 1978.

Nutrition Information Resources for the Whole Family. National Nutrition Education Clearing House, 1978.

Nutrition Labeling: How It Can Work for You. National Nutrition Consortium, American Dietetic Association, 1975.

Nutrition Source Book. Rosemont, IL: Nationary Dairy Council, 1978.

*Passnater, Richard A. Super Nutrition. New York: Dial, 1975.

*Pauling, Linus. Vitamin C and the Common Cold. New York: Bantam Books, 1971.

Piltz, Albert. How Your Body Uses Food. Rosemont, IL: National Dairy Council, 1960.

*Pommery, Jean. *What to Do till the Veterinarian Comes*. Radnor, PA: Chilton Book Company, 1976.

"Present Knowledge in Nutrition." *Nutrition Reviews*. Nutrition Foundation, Inc., 1976.

*Rodale, J.I. *The Complete Book of Minerals for Health*. 4th ed. Emmaus, PA: Rodale Books, 1976.

*————. *The Encyclopedia of Common Diseases*. Emmaus, PA: Rodale Press, 1976.

*Rosenberg, Harold, and Feldzaman, A.N. *Doctor's Book of Vitamin Therapy: Megavitamins for Health*. New York: Putnam's, 1974.

*Seamen, Barbara and Gideon. *Women and the Crisis in Sex Hormones*. New York: Rawson Associates Publishers, 1977.

*Shute, Wilfrid E., and Taub, Harold J. *Vitamin E for Ailing and Healthy Hearts*. New York: Pyramid Books, 1969.

*Spock, Benjamin. *Baby and Child Care*. New York: Simon and Schuster, 1976.

"Too Much Sugar." *Consumer Reports* 43 (March 1978).

Underwood, Eric J. *Trace Elements in Human and Animal Nutrition*. 4th ed. New York: Academic Press, 1977.

United Nations. Food and Agriculture Organization. *Calorie Requirements*, 1957, 1972.

U.S. Department of Agriculture. *Amino Acid Content of Food* by M.L. Orr and B.K. Watt, 1957; rev. 1968.

U.S. Department of Agriculture. Consumer and Food Economics Institute, Agricultural Research Service. *Composition of Foods: Raw, Processed, Prepared* by Bernice K. Watt and Annabel L. Merrill, 1975.

U.S. Department of Agriculture. *Energy Value of Foods: Basis and Derivation* by Annabel L. Merrill and Bernice K. Watt, 1973.

U.S. Department of Agriculture. *Nutritive Value of American Foods* by Catherine F. Adams, 1975.

U.S. Department of Health, Education and Welfare. *Consumer Health Education: A Directory*, 1975.

U.S. Department of Health, Education and Welfare.

Ten-State Nutrition Survey. Washington, DC: U.S. Government Printing Office, 1968–70.

"The U.S. Food and Drug Administration: On Food and Drugs." *Consumer Reports* 38 (March 1973).

U.S. President's Council on Physical Fitness and Sports. *Exercise and Weight Control* by Robert E. Johnson. Urbana, IL: Univ. of Illinois Press, 1967.

U.S. Senate. Select Committee on Nutrition and Human Needs. *Diet and Killer Diseases with Press Reaction and Additional Information.* Washington, DC: U.S. Government Printing Office, 1977.

U.S. Senate. Select Committee on Nutrition and Human Needs. *National Nutrition Policy: Nutrition and the Consumer II.* Washington, DC: U.S. Government Printing Office, 1974.

"Vitamin-Mineral Safety, Toxicity and Misuse." *Journal of the American Dietetic Association,* 1978.

*Wade, Carlson. *Magic Minerals.* West Nyack, NY: Parker Publishing Co., 1967.

*———. *Miracle Protein.* West Nyack, NY: Parker Publishing Co., 1975.

*———. *Vitamin E: The Rejuvenation Vitamin.* New York: Award Books, 1970.

"Which Cereals Are Most Nutritious?" *Consumer Reports* 40 (February 1975).

Williams, Roger J. *Nutrition Against Disease.* New York: Pitman Publishers, 1971.

*Winter, Ruth. *A Consumer's Dictionary of Food Additives.* New York: Crown, 1978.

*Young, Klein, Beyer. *Recreational Drugs.* New York: Macmillan, 1977.

*Yudkin, John. *Sweet and Dangerous.* New York: Peter H. Wyden, 1972.

Index

341

342

343

347

348